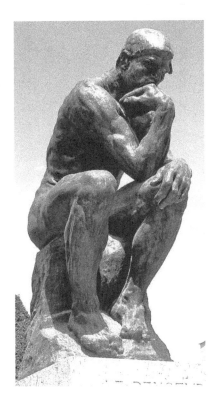

If one of us must be cast in bronze
Let it not be the fading, in anguish
Nor the thinker, in silent contemplation
Let it be the fallen, in reverence.
Zachary Gospe, 2015

We Can,
But Should We?

*One Physician's Reflections on
End of Life Ethical Dilemmas*

J. Michael Gospe, M.D.

Copyright © 2016

By

J. Michael Gospe, M.D.

*******ISBN <978-1-5306-2584-0>********

J. Michael Gospe, M.D.
1701 Pamela Drive
Santa Rosa, CA 95404
Email: mgospe@sonic.net.
https://gospemedicalethics.wordpress.com/home/

To
John William "Jack" Glaser (1933-2012)
&
Corrine Bayley

For their
unique insights into human behavior
&
guidance in my learning the art of medical ethics.

And to
Allen Barbour, M.D. (1918-1993)

For teaching me to
"Always be gentle with your patients.
They are people, not just diseases."

Acknowledgements

This book has taken forty-six years of gestation. I could not do this Herculean task without many midwives in the delivery room before words formed on my computer screen.

I am deeply indebted to the patients and staff of Santa Rosa Memorial Hospital. I am especially grateful to David, Diane, Edwin, Jennifer, Jose, Kristan, Lucille, Paul, Satero, Tyree, and many other patients whose stories fill these pages.

Rebecca Bondhus-Calley has been my close companion and strategist over twenty years. Together we have led our two hospital ethics committees: the Medical Ethics Resource Service and the Ethics Coordinating Council. I wish to thank the members of these committees, the leaders of similar groups within the St. Joseph of Orange hospital community, and the Vice Presidents of Theology and Ethics of St. Joseph of Orange extending from Jack Glaser in 1982 through David C. Blake, Johnny Cox, Kevin Murphy, to Daniel Dwyer today. I also thank Corrine Bayley, Barbara Cox, and Jennifer Dunatov for their roles in helping me during their time at St. Joseph of Orange's Department of Theology and Ethics. Gary Johanson, M.D. and Andrew Wagner, M.D. have been especially helpful with their indepth insights of complex cases that we have had in common.

This work would not have been brought into the light of day without Sam Kimbles' persistence in reminding me that my experiences in medical ethics needed to be shared with others.

Thanks to Clara Rosemarda and her *Creative Writing Workshops* where I am challenged to dig into my subconscious to release hidden truths with pen to page. Thanks also to our monthly afternoon writing group of Anne Marie Cheney, Gerry Gospe, Karen Miller, and myself who repeatedly critiqued my rough drafts.

Webmaster, J. Michael Gospe, Jr., established my webpage at http://gospemedicalethics.wordpress.com/home/. I have unbounded appreciation for his efforts and experience. He also helped shape the book's final cover.

J. Michael Gospe, M.D.

My grandson, Zachary Gospe, continues to awe me with his poem, *The Thinker*. He elegantly captured the theme of this book in a handful of words.

I give special thanks to my family of involved editors. My brother, Stephen Gospe, M.D., saw that the medical information and grammar made sense. My daughter, Kathy Parnay, pushed me toward deeper thinking to expand my thoughts.

Finally, I am most grateful to my wife, Gerry Gospe, who has spent uncountable hours reviewing my work. Her experiences as a wife of over fifty-five years, mother of five, public health nurse, and spiritual director have given her valuable insights into the ethical dilemmas I face in the hospital. She has the uncanny ability to transform rambling sentences into smooth phrases as she simplifies and condenses my scattered words into a cohesive whole.

Contents

Acknowledgements vii

Preface 1

Chapter 1: Living Life on the Edge 4
 (Autonomy)

Chapter 2: Changing Image 11
 (Beneficence)

Chapter 3: Not a Leg to Stand On 19
 (Non-maleficence)

Chapter 4: The Shadow Side 26
 (Justice)

Chapter 5: The Small Card 34
 (Fidelity)

Chapter 6: Kitty Cats 42
 (Goals of Therapy)

Chapter 7: Window of Opportunity 49
 (Capacity)

Chapter 8: Who's on First? 56
 (Surrogacy)

Chapter 9: "Listen to Me!" 64
 (Advance Health Care Directive)

Chapter 10: No Man is an Island   70
    (Communication)

Chapter 11: "I Love My Son"   78
    (Case Conferences)

Chapter 12: Waiting …   89
    (Cultural Conflicts)

Chapter 13: "Let Me Go!"   97
    (Hydration and Nutrition)

Chapter 14: Out of the Box   104
    (Non-compliance)

Chapter 15: Inevitable Death   112
    (Miracles)

Chapter 16: Home?   120
    (Access to Care)

Chapter 17: Further Reflections   127
    (Dignity, Informed Consent, Active Listening)

Chapter 18: The Last Word   137

About the Author   140

Preface

I'm not certain if bioethics chose me, or if I chose bioethics. It doesn't really matter. The important thing is that it changed me in ways I could not imagine when I volunteered to join my hospital's bioethics group at their second meeting in 1982.

By that time, I had been practicing gastroenterology and internal medicine for over a decade. I had accompanied numerous patients during the final stages of their life. My intuition told me I needed to learn more about the dying process itself and the tapestry it weaves between patients, families, and caregivers. I find this work as compelling, challenging, and invigorating today as when I first began my medical practice over forty-five years ago.

Conflicts can and do occur between the values of patients, family members, and staff. Early intervention is crucial before stress levels increase so that communication between all parties becomes nearly impossible. For this reason, multi-faceted case conferences continue to invite all folks, professional and lay alike, to voice concerns and to plan strategies. One of the most difficult examples of such a conflict would be when a surrogate or physician must go against the desires of the patient's family in order to follow the patient's wishes. This is especially common when considering the discontinuation of curative medical treatment and moving into comfort care. Another example would be when a surrogate fails to act according to the patient's expressed wishes or best interest. Conflicts like these complicate

1

solving medical dilemmas by adding heightened emotions that can jeopardize optimal patient care.

A dilemma always presents two or more possible solutions to a problem. Each response contains a conflicting set of benefits and burdens. I liken a medical ethical dilemma to a broken ancient pottery urn. When I first look on the pieces that litter the ground, my eyes see a multitude of small irregular unrelated shapes. It may take hours of struggle to find where each one fits. When all folks involved can lay out their bits and pieces of information, we see a broader view that illustrates the pros and cons of each solution. The urn takes form as we witness the shards morph into a beautiful vessel in the shape of possibility. Most of all, it can foster a heartfelt peace in us. Our patient is receiving the best of care for her condition according to her desires.

A peaceful aura surrounds a patient who accepts that she is living her last days with her family close by. I have noticed the cohesive bonding that enfolds the patient when loved ones, caregivers, and hospital personnel work with the patient as an active participant.

I've learned that patience is important. It may be necessary to repeat gently and simply the benefits and burdens of each treatment. It is a way to engender trust, support, and care for the patient and family.

The practice of medicine entrusts physicians and staff to find appropriate medical solutions to best meet their patients' hopes and desires. In this way, they serve patients, their families, and the hospital community according to the values set before them. There is wisdom to be gleaned when the team of medical personnel and family members share their concerns, doubts, and grief as they travel this part of life's journey. I am being constantly enriched by our common engagement. I believe others are too.

I wrote *We Can, But Should We? One Physician's Reflections on End of Life Ethical Dilemmas* for healthcare workers, patients, and families. The book explores medical ethical dilemmas in a hospital setting. It offers a path through a complex maze when we enter the realm of *we can—but should we?* This book will alert you to potential ethical problems that might be developing right now or in the future. You will become

WE CAN, BUT SHOULD WE?

familiar with the nature of an ethical dilemma. Included are some tools to identify proactive ways in seeking resolution of complex issues before they grow into unmanageable situations.

I invite you to look at these sixteen stories as stepping-stones towards forming your own goals when you find yourself in similar quandaries. Each one has taught me about the frailty and strength in being human. I have altered names and events to protect the privacy of my patients and the staff. Individual chapters relate to a specific ethical value. I hope they will offer you new ways to approach issues that arise at the end of life.

My heartfelt wish is that you will be moved to talk to your family and friends about your own wishes while you are enjoying life. It is never too early; it is never too late.

J. Michael Gospe, M.D.
2016

You can find more information on these topics at my website: http://gospemedicalethics.wordpress.com/home/.

1
Living Life on the Edge
Autonomy

Clyde Anderson is seventy-eight. He has severe neurological injuries from a motorcycle-truck accident. The physicians want to change the goal of treatment to comfort care. There is some hostility among the staff when Mrs. Anderson insists upon intensive active therapy. It is unclear what Mr. Anderson would want.

It is a foggy Friday morning, a perfect day for writing, when the phone rings. Its Caller I.D. reads *Memorial Hospital*. I answer with a smile, a far different response from the time when I was in solo private practice. In those days, the calls demanded an immediate trip to the emergency room to diagnose and treat patients with a GI bleed or liver failure. During those five-minute races to the hospital, my adrenal glands spewed adrenaline as my mind sifted through a fast forward film of possible scenarios that might meet me.

Now, ten retirement years later, I greet the calls with relaxed curiosity. A request for an ethical consultation usually involves end of life issues. They require me to listen with care; to familiarize myself with patients, family, and staff; and to note questions that arise from gathered information. I find that in a conference-like atmosphere, we can dissect complex dilemmas into options, diffuse confusion, and discover appropriate care for the patient.

WE CAN, BUT SHOULD WE?

I relish time: time to evaluate and offer a plan for a conversation; time to present the patient's current status; time to invite all voices to speak. This is one of those cases.

Mark Boynton is on the line. He is a seasoned nurse in the intensive care unit and is calling for a consultation. I reach for a pen and a pad of paper, ready for his story.

"The Trauma Team admitted a seventy-eight year-old man whose motorbike was T-boned by a truck a week ago. The poor guy suffered severe brain damage. It's clear to the docs that he'll never recover from his injuries. The neurosurgeon doubts he'll regain consciousness. His vitals are dropping and his brain is herniating." Mark pauses for a second. "We all want to stop the pressers, remove the respirator, and emphasize comfort care."

"Sounds reasonable. What's the ethical issue?"

"His wife is adamant about continuing with everything. She's not able to take in what the docs tell her: that her husband is dying and can't be saved."

"What's your patient's name and room number? I'll pop by the hospital to review his records and take a look at him. I'll call you when I have more data."

"Thanks, Mike. His name is Clyde Anderson. He's located in ICU East, Room 252."

"I should be able to get back to you within an hour."

As I look through Mr. Anderson's history, a comment made by the doctor who admitted him strikes me. *Mr. Anderson was one of the founders of a Hell's Angel motorcycle group in San Francisco in the 1960's. He still rides a motorcycle.*

My mind flashes back to my medical residency years in San Francisco when my training all but buried me. Even though I lived in the edge of the Haight-Ashbury District at the time, my major contact with that scene was through television images of flower children, drugs, antiwar riots, and motorcycle groups. I immediately imagine a gang of men dressed in black leather pants and jackets emblazoned with Hell's Angels' emblems as they hog the road with revving engines. I wonder what my personal contact with this Hell's Angel will be like.

5

J. Michael Gospe, M.D.

Before the accident, Mr. Anderson's general health was excellent with the exception of some mild blood pressure elevation. He and several friends were riding their motorcycles along the narrow winding costal Highway 1, north of Jenner. A loaded truck struck him as it was rolling down the steep hill he was climbing. It took twenty minutes for the medical helicopter to arrive at the scene. The first responders found Mr. Anderson non-responsive with difficulty breathing. He had a severe head injury and multiple fractured bones.

Our neurosurgeon met Mr. Anderson in the emergency room and immediately brought him to surgery where the patient underwent burr hole placement to relieve pressure on his brain. During the eleven days of his hospitalization, Mr. Anderson's health deteriorated.

Presently, he is receiving ventilator support, intravenous fluids, and medications to keep his blood and central nervous system pressures in near normal range. When I call the trauma doctor of the day, the neurosurgeon, and the intensivist, each one agrees that Mr. Anderson's prognosis for recovery is nil. None of them consider active treatment appropriate. Each doctor recommends a transition to comfort care. The intensivist laments, "We are beating the man to death with our treatments while his wife is pushing us to continue to do everything we can. She doesn't understand we are unable to make him better."

I return my call to Mark Boynton with my summary. "Mark. It seems to me that the best approach for Mr. Anderson would be to set up a meeting with Mrs. Anderson, her support group, his physicians, his primary nurse, and a chaplain. Hopefully, when the family and staff discuss Mr. Anderson's condition together, it may be possible for his wife and doctors to arrive at a mutually acceptable plan of action. The social worker will contact the family and team for a meeting tomorrow at eleven in the ICU Conference Room."

I arrive early at the small conference room and place the chairs in circular fashion. A box of tissues sits on a small end table for those tearful moments that are sure to come during this somber meeting.

The staff, Mrs. Anderson, and three of her friends arrive and take their seats. I look at the men who come with her and feel my heartbeats convert into flight mode. The men tower over my five feet six inch frame and one hundred forty pounds. I estimate each man being seven feet tall and weighing over three hundred pounds of pure muscle. In my mind they appear to sport a week's growth of beard covering a snarly face with pointed teeth. Black leather jackets with stenciled slogans on the back drape over one of each of their hairy tattoo-covered arms. Dirty tee shirts cover their potbellies. One of them has a package of Lucky Strikes rolled up in his left short sleeve. Am I intimidated? You bet.

For a moment, I lose my calm. I imagine that verbal and physical abuse will overrun the next hour. I picture a long string of motorcycles roaring down Highway 1, weaving in and out of traffic and squeezing all of the car and truck drivers in their way to the edge of the road.

I break my momentary trance with several deep breaths to calm myself back into the present moment. As we introduce ourselves and I look each person eye to eye, I feel a sense of our common goal. We are here for Mr. Anderson, our loved one, our friend, and our patient. I invite Mrs. Anderson to share her understanding about her husband's goals in life, his current status, and the expected outcome of his disease.

Mrs. Anderson tells us that she and her husband recently celebrated their fortieth wedding anniversary. From their very beginning, she knew he lived his life on the edge; he thrived on taking chances. Mr. Anderson loved driving his bike off-road at high speeds, feeling the wind blow through his hair. When he was a young man he smoked, shot, and snorted any drug he could get his hands on. During the 60's and 70's he was in and out of jail, generally for disturbing the peace. He was never a member of an organized religion and did not believe in a supreme being. On the other hand, he has a strong sense of joy in life, an aspect that makes up an integral part of his psyche. Mrs. Anderson is certain that her husband would want to continue all forms of active treatment until he breathes his last breath. Comfort care is not for him. His goal is to live as long as possible.

After a pause, the physicians explain the results of their findings in simple terms. Each of them repeats the fact that active care is no longer a benefit for Mr. Anderson's body; he is in his last hours or days.

Finally, I open up the discussion to the motorcycle club and the rest of the staff. Mr. Anderson's motorcycle buddies are surprisingly articulate and polite. They had nodded their agreement with much of what Mrs. Anderson said as she talked about her husband.

Their grief around the loss of their long-time friend is visible. They listened carefully to what the physicians say. One man speaks about how his companion formed their motorcycle club years before he was born.

I find myself surprised as my one-dimensional caricature of members of motorcycle gang members gradually morphs into a living, breathing Mr. Anderson. He is a man who had formed an indelible bond with the three men in front of me. I am moved by the love and respect that Mr. Anderson's wife and companions have for him.

I see the members of the hospital staff relax in their chairs as their frustration moves to understanding. It's not that Mrs. Anderson doesn't listen to the doctors or that she doesn't understand the situation. Actually, it is just the opposite. She lives in the hope her husband will rally. At the same time she knows her husband wants to ride his bike to the end of this road, wherever it leads.

Although this is not what any of us expected, there is unanimous agreement among the physicians: active treatment will continue based upon Mrs. Anderson's knowledge of her husband. He would likely agree with the current proactive approach to his care. At the same time, we arrange for a follow-up meeting in five days to reconsider Mr. Anderson's condition and the medical treatment we will offer to him.

We never have that second meeting. Although all the medications and treatment continue, they do not reverse Mr. Anderson's downward spiral. He passes away the next afternoon. He dies the way he lived, the way he wanted: his throttle on high and his wheels burning rubber.

Reflections

Autonomy

Autonomy is the value of self-determination. It respects the patient by enabling him to be the ultimate judge of what is to happen to his body. The coherent patient is the only one who can best understand the benefits and burdens of any medical treatment offered to him. This is self-determination at its fullest. If he is unable to speak for himself then it is the obligation of the staff and surrogate to attempt to discover what he would have chosen for himself.

Mr. Anderson's story presents a typical medical dilemma emanating from the downward spiral of his condition despite intense medical treatment. A serious disagreement between Mr. Anderson's family and the staff about the goals of therapy threatened to interfere with his care. The case conference allowed all parties to balance opposing options and focus on qualities that were most important to Mr. Anderson.

As health care professionals, it is important for us to keep our own personal beliefs and judgments to ourselves, lest we overpower those of the patient or his family. Life is complex and affects us in different ways. Each of us has unique experiences that form our thoughts about our life and our eventual death. When we ponder our own meaning in life, we enter the spiritual realm. Whether we are an atheist, an agnostic, a member of an established body of faith, or do not claim a particular belief, in dying we are faced with our finite ending as we know it. In this place of surrender, we bring the sum of who we are in the present moment: our values, our purpose, and our deepest desires.

Our hospitals consist of microcosms of the world around us. Visitors, patients, and staff walk the corridors. Among them are first and second generation Chinese, Hmong, Eritrean, Central American, and Filipino, to name a few. We have contact with patients who are homeless and those living in estates, alcoholics and abstainers, drug users, policemen, grocers, executives, and members of motorcycle gangs. An error we professionals can easily fall into is to assume that all people who are of the same heritage or life style agree about life and death. When we profile someone, we lose sight of him/her as an individual. This is a grave mistake.

J. Michael Gospe, M.D.

If it is difficult to put our own beliefs into words without deep thought, it is infinitely more difficult to intuit the beliefs held by another[1]. It is important to remember that a vulnerable person, especially in a hospital setting, will struggle to find ways to express his feelings. Perhaps these might be some questions to raise with our patients who know they are actively dying:

- *How are you faring today?*
- *Is there unfinished business you need to attend to?*
- *What do you hold dear at this moment?*
- *In the time you have left, what would you most want to accomplish?*

We need to discuss these issues with our loved ones when we are alert, to inform them about our values and desires. Often a newspaper article, a television show, a movie, or an event that affected a friend may be a perfect segue to begin a conversation on end of life issues.

I recommend that adults of any age complete an Advance Health Care Document[2] when in good health.

- *Discuss your views with persons close to you.*
- *Select a surrogate.*
- *Take the document out and review it periodically as circumstances change.*
- *Keep several copies handy.*

---

1. Chapter 12: *Waiting* ... (Cultural Differences)
2. Chapter 9: *"Listen to Me!"* (Advance Health Care Document)

2
Changing Image
Beneficence

Sally Reins is nineteen. She is severely disabled and has recurrent pneumonia due to difficulty in swallowing. A consultant recommended major surgery to prevent further aspiration of her stomach contents. Her pediatrician is concerned that surgery may not be in her best interest.

Bill, a pediatrician, is a large man of fifty-one. He resembles a teddy bear with a perpetual smile. This particular morning we cross paths while waiting for an elevator in the hospital.

"Mike. Do you have a moment to talk?"

"Oh. Hi, Bill. Good to see you. What's up?"

"I need your help as the Ethics' Chair. I don't know if I have a problem or not, but I'm feeling concerned about one of my patients."

I nod and Bill takes a deep breath. "I have a severely disabled girl in Pediatrics. This is her third hospitalization in six months for a recurrent pneumonia. She keeps vomiting gastric acid into her lungs. I'm worried about her frequent aspirations."

He smiles. "Sally was one of my first patients; she's nineteen now. She has lived with her caretaker, Frieda, for over fifteen years. Sally is precious and Frieda is a saint the way she cares for her." He went on, "Yesterday, I obtained a pulmonary consultation. Although my consultant's recommendation appears relatively simple, I'm uncomfortable with his plan. It seems that the best way to prevent further damage to Sally's lungs is to have her undergo three surgical procedures. He wants to close off the upper part of her stomach to prevent vomiting, place a feeding tube through her abdominal wall to feed her, and give her a tracheotomy to prevent her saliva from flowing into her lungs."

As Bill tells me Sally's story, he begins to slowly rub his hands together as if he were massaging his thoughts. "I can't put it into words, but I feel the surgery might not be in Sally's best interests. I ran it by one of the surgeons who said the surgery would be straightforward and she should fly through it." Bill inhales slowly and sighs, "Mike, will you please take a look at Sally for me? I know the surgeries would eliminate her aspirating, but something tells me it's not the right thing to do."

In my mind, I agree with Bill's consultants. However, something intangible troubles him, something that would not allow him to send Sally to surgery without more thought. Bill relaxes and a grin comes to his face when I say, "I'll look into it right away. I'll get back to you later today."

I visit Sally before reading her chart. I am touched by Bill's calling her *precious*. I find her room quiet. At first, I think the nurses transferred her elsewhere. A silent television hangs from the ceiling, its screen dark. A small table, next to a gray steel-lined electrical bed, holds a blue plastic pitcher with matching cup, a small box of facial tissues, and a phone.

Then my eyes wander to the bed where I notice a form. Sally looks like an emaciated doll. A thin white sheet covers her motionless figure. I look closer. Her twisted arms and legs curl into a tight fetal position. She doesn't look as if she weighs over 35 pounds. At that moment, a picture of a child imprisoned in a concentration camp comes to mind. I gaze at her face. Two open, but unfocused, green eyes stare into space.

With this likeness imprinted in my mind, I leave Sally's room for the nurses' station to review her hospital records. I read in the physician's notes that she was born with cerebral palsy and a severe genetic disorder, Trisomy 18. These conditions resulted in a combination of untreatable neuromuscular abnormalities, mental retardation, and cardiac defects.

WE CAN, BUT SHOULD WE?

Over the nearly two decades of her life, Sally's mind remained that of an infant. She required twenty-four hour care. The only part of her body she could move was her left arm, slightly, without obvious purpose. She could not speak; she communicated by occasional grunts and groans. Her current pneumonia was healing with antibiotics. She would be ready for discharge in several days unless she was to undergo surgery.

The hospital social worker reported in the chart that Frieda's license to be a caregiver only allowed her to look after uncomplicated patients. If Sally were to have either a tracheotomy or feeding tube, she would have to leave Frieda's home for a more skilled facility. Unfortunately, there were none nearby. At discharge from our hospital, she would need to transfer to a large skilled nursing facility for handicapped patients in another county. The social worker also wrote that Sally's parents were divorced a number of years ago and her mother is no longer involved with Sally. Sally's father visits her monthly and takes her to his home every Christmas. He would have difficulty visiting his daughter if she moved away from the area.

I can now see Bill's dilemma. Surgery would be a mechanical approach to an anatomic problem: the presence of recurrent stomach acid invading Sally's lungs resulting in repeated episodes of pneumonia. Accepting surgery would offer her a chance for a longer life without the risk of further lung disease. However, the surgery would also require separation and loss of support from her loved ones as well as a change from her familiar surroundings.

Later in the day, I return to Sally's room and am surprised to see that the afternoon sun now streams through the windows. It creates a warm glow throughout the formerly dark space. A small glass vase overflows with fresh red and white roses and decorates the bedside table. A comedy is playing on the television; its soft volume brings a sign of life to the once quiet environment.

A rotund fifty year-old woman with a glowing aura surrounding her face sits on the side of the hospital bed. She gently brushes Sally's long red tresses, spread over her shrunken chest. I guess she is Frieda, Sally's caregiver, surrogate mother, and friend of fifteen years.

J. Michael Gospe, M.D.

"Hi, I'm Dr. Gospe; you must be Frieda. Sally's doctor asked me to drop in and look at her. Would you mind telling me a bit about Sally?"

"Sally's a sweetheart, Doctor. The other three girls in my house love her. They're not as disabled as Sally and talk to her as they play games and watch TV. They were heartbroken when the ambulance took Sally to the hospital the other day. They can't wait to have her home again." Frieda adds, "My aide and I get Sally up between 8:00 and 9:00 in the morning. After we clean and dress her, we put her in a special chair for the day." Frieda's lips formed a lovely smile as she continues, "When the weather is warm, Sally enjoys sitting in the sun in the back yard where she can watch the other girls in the sandbox. Her three great loves in life are having her hair brushed, eating the soft foods we feed her, and cooing with us." Frieda looks at Sally and reaches for a tissue as her eyes begin to glisten. Slowly, with a great deal of emotion, she continues, "Sally understands us, she loves us and we love her. I wouldn't want anything bad to ever happen to my little girl."

As I gaze at Sally, I wonder if this is really the same person I saw a few hours ago. It is as if a magician had uttered unpronounceable words after covering her tiny body with multicolored silk. When he whipped back the psychedelic material, a new likeness of the young woman appeared. There are similarities; however, enough differences exist making me suspect that either my perspective is altered or a doppelgänger of Sally now occupies the bed.

I fuse the two impressions into one picture: that of a severely handicapped patient with a deteriorating body and that of a human being able to receive and radiate love. I realize the truth exists somewhere between the death-like image of my first view and the very ill, angelic young lady who lies in front of me. Sally's cooing and babbling interact with Frieda's quiet touches. Clean, without sores or bruises, Sally's skin reveals evidence of many years of attention and care. It is immediately obvious to me that a close, communicative relationship radiates between the two of them.

At that moment I remember an optical illusion I first saw when I was ten years old. The picture was a fusion of two faces with a caption reading, "Do you see the face of an old woman or a pretty young lady?" When I first viewed the drawing, it took several minutes before I was able to identify each of the faces. Once I found them, I had difficulty in focusing on only one at a time. The images seemed to drift into and out of each other, as does the ebb and flow of the tide onto a sandy beach at the ocean's edge. So it was as I ponder the two visions I had of Sally.

I realize that both Bill and Sally's father needed more information concerning the choices available for Sally. I arrange a meeting between them and the staff caring for her. I hope that creative thinking during this session will clarify the best goals for Sally and how to achieve them.

The next afternoon, ten of us meet. During an hour of sensitive and informative discussion, the powerful bond of love that exists between Sally and Frieda strike all of us around the table. We learn about Sally's quality of life, her relationships with the other handicapped girls in Frieda's care, and the affection Sally's father has toward his daughter. This quiet girl who could never speak ignites a light within my heart.

As the meeting proceeds, we consider how surgery would affect her. She would not be able to swallow food or vocalize sounds, two of her greatest enjoyments in life. We feel that a move away from her home and into a large care facility would diminish Sally's personal and constant care. Moreover it would create a wrenching loss for her father and Frieda. We deem that the burdens of the suggested surgery's results are inappropriate for Sally's situation. Sally's father decides to refuse surgery.

Now we are left with finding a plan that would allow Sally to remain with Frieda. Our concern revolves around Sally developing repeated pneumonia. What happens if she requires more complicated treatment beyond what Frieda's care license permits?

Fortunately, several representatives of the county organization overseeing Sally's care are with us. Agreeing with the determination to have Sally return to Frieda's home, the agency bends the rules that did not allow Frieda to care for a dying client. This makes it possible for Frieda to keep Sally for the remainder of her life.

Three years later, I meet Frieda at another care conference. My heart leaps when she tells me Sally is still with her and has not had another bout of pneumonia. Clearly, Sally's father and her physician made the proper decision on that day of uncertainty when a discussion of benefits and burdens by a caring group helped solve a medical dilemma.

Reflections

Beneficence

Beneficence is the value of doing *good* for another person. It teams up with non-maleficence[1], *do no harm*. I look at these values as being two sides of the same coin. Therapeutic treatment may contain both good and harm from the patient's perspective. Most importantly, it must fit the patient's needs and desires whenever possible. When the options do not fit the patient, then it is time to seek other solutions.

Sally's metamorphosis continues to affect the way I observe a patient. My first impression is just that. Sally came alive when Frieda arrived; the sound of her voice, her familiar touch, and her care of the environment brought life into the room. The lesson for me is to remember there is always more beneath my first observation. Now I look for clues beyond the external snapshot. What was this person's life like? Her joys? Her sorrows? Just like my optical illusion of the old woman, there hides an internal beauty. Sally's two images merge into one whole being.

The benefits and burdens of planned treatment hold contrasting and complex issues that stretch beyond employing a specific procedure or medication. There are no guaranteed outcomes. If a treatment or operation has an 85% chance of success, the first thought is that its good outweighs its burdens. We must never forget that the same statistic means there is a 15% chance of failure with its own scenario.

An example of this might be the recommendation of experimental therapy for an aggressive cancer. Its advantage could be the hope of improving life expectancy by weeks or even several months. It is up to the patient or surrogate to consider the possible good results with the suffering and lasting effects that may occur from the treatment itself.

WE CAN, BUT SHOULD WE?

How would a chosen therapy affect the quality of the patient's remaining life? Is it time to shift to comfort care to relieve the patient's pain and suffering? Is it time for her to take a long-wished trip to Tahiti? I shall never forget Horace, a patient of mine who against medical advise opted to forgo a liver transplant for his biliary cirrhosis and spend his last few weeks at his beloved cabin in the High Sierras.

Here are a few important questions for the patient, family, and staff to take into consideration:

- *What does she need/want in her dying process?*
- *How would the suggested treatment and its side effects affect her quality of life?*
- *Are there other alternatives to her planned treatment?*
- *Are funds available to provide her extended care?*
- *How does she live her life? In fear? Alone?*
- *Is she a hopeful person?*
- *What are her spiritual or religious beliefs?*
- *Does she have a supporting community?*
- *What does she need to prepare for her death?*

The answer to all of these queries is that *it all depends* on what the situation reveals at any given moment. These decisions are hard to make for oneself. It is much more difficult to do so for a loved one, and nearly impossible to make for a patient whom you do not intimately know. Yet, these are situations in which each one of us who cares for a dying patient may find ourselves. Time, thought, and sharing with others helps to crystalize the enigmas we often face in medicine.

Finally, keep in mind to listen to your patient's, her surrogate's, and her loved one's questions. Answer as honestly as possible. Try to arrange family members or clergy to be present when discussing life-threatening issues. Give them time to absorb the information, time to ask more questions, even if it means returning for another meeting.

One of the hardest lessons I had to learn over and over again during my medical practice was how to separate my own desires *for* my patient from those *of* my patient. The important lesson here is that the individual patient's perspective must determine the quality of beneficence. My role is to help my patient, family, and surrogate to understand the choices presented and to support their final decision.

J. Michael Gospe, M.D.

In Chapter 1, *Living Life on the Edge*, all of the caregivers had strong feelings about the appropriateness of intensive therapy for Clyde Anderson. A simple gathering of family, friends, and staff taught us about his life style and probable preference for continued active care. Fortunately, his physicians and nurses listened to, and understood, what those who knew Mr. Anderson were saying about the way he lived his seventy-eight years.

In our current chapter, we were unable to rely on Sally or her history to determine her wishes because of Sally's severe birth disabilities. Yet, we observed a sustainable quality of life through Sally's intimate ways of relating to her caregiver. Surgery would strip away Sally's loving and supporting community. Our conference gathered as a *community of concern*[2] consisting of family, caregivers, staff, and physicians to develop a plan that would be in her best interests, one that would promote her well being in accordance with respect for her dignity[3].

---

1. Chapter 3: *Not a Leg to Stand On* (Non-Maleficence)
2. *Community of concern* is a term coined by Jack Glaser describing a multidisciplinary group of members of the medical, paramedical, and family who are intimately involved with the patient and are brought together to focus on the needs of a specific patient.
3. Chapter 17: *Further Reflections* (Dignity)

3
Not a Leg to Stand On
Non-maleficence

Carol Juleps is a forty-four year-old woman who took an overdose of sedatives. She lay in a twisted position for over twenty-four hours. The weight of her body compromised the blood flow to her lower extremities. Her surgeon wants to amputate both legs but her family refuses to give permission for the operation.

I am in my usual morning rush. After completing my hospital rounds, I hurry over to the Doctors' Lounge to collect my daily portion of unending reports and memos that fill my pigeonholed mailbox. I only have a few minutes before I need to be at the Outpatient Surgical Department when I feel a tap on my shoulder.

Ted Brock, a general surgeon, captures my attention with his clenched teeth and wrinkled brow. "Mike. Can you help me with an ethics consultation?"

"Sure, Ted. What's up?"

"I've got a gal, Carol Juleps, in the surgical unit. She took an overdose a couple of weeks ago. The next morning, her daughter, Debra, discovered her lying in a heap on the bedroom floor. The weight of her twisted trunk pinched her femoral arteries and decreased the blood supply to the muscles of her left thigh and right calf. The resulting gangrene caused her to develop kidney failure. She is now on dialysis. I've already performed three surgical procedures to remove dead and damaged tissue from her legs. She's going to die if I don't take off her legs pretty darn soon."

"What's keeping you from operating?"

"It's her family. Momma won't say much, but Debra is angry and impossible to talk to. Seems like all she wants is for her mother to die and get out of her hair. To make matters worse, Carol's psychiatrist and her primary care physician are both on vacation and we can't reach them."

"Ted, your patient's name seems familiar. I'll check my office records before I see her."

When I pull Carol's chart, I find it has been three years since I have seen her. At that time, her psychiatrist asked me to evaluate her chronic abdominal pain. My notes read in part: *extremely anxious and depressed thirty-nine year old lady with numerous inconsistent complaints of constipation, diarrhea, and non-specific abdominal pain.* My workup included an extensive history and physical examination, lab work, and endoscopies to evaluate her stomach and colon. The findings suggested that her problem was an irritable bowel syndrome. She failed to keep her scheduled follow-up office appointment. I did not see her again.

After lunch, I peruse Carol's current hospital record. Although she woke up two days after her admission, she was intermittently confused with little understanding of her condition. Her physicians were certain that amputation of both legs, the left above the knee and the right below the knee, would be necessary to save her life.

I speak with Carol's primary nurse who tells me Carol suffers from a debilitating chronic depression. This agrees with my earlier findings. The nurse goes on to say, "Even though the gangrenous smell makes changing her dressings a nightmare, most of us feel that amputating both of her legs would be devastating for her and severely deepen her depression. Some of the nurses are upset that the doctor is even talking to the family about surgery."

I speak to Rachel, the social worker assigned to the surgical unit. She tells me, "Carol's mother and daughter come to the hospital on a daily basis. Her mother is usually quiet and weepy. On the other hand, Debra is belligerent and angry. She faults nearly every aspect of her mother's hospital care from diet to roommate to the noise level in the hallway. She tells everyone that her mother must be allowed to die. Her explosive behavior affects everyone: the patient, the family, and the staff."

An overwhelming odor of decaying flesh meets me as I stand at the threshold of Carol's room. I gulp down an eruption of acid that arises from my stomach and wait for the heaving motion within me to subside. I remember a patient I cared for as an intern over twenty years ago. He was an elderly diabetic with a decaying leg. The same stench of gangrene surrounded him as he took his last breath.

I don a thick yellow isolation gown and protective rubber gloves to prevent me from collecting and spreading the many strains of bacteria swimming in Carol's wounds.

Although only forty-four, Carol's malnourished body makes her look much older. A short hospital gown covers the upper part of her bony body. She is semiconscious and moans with pain. A heat lamp beams drying rays onto the extensive rotting tissues of her legs. I see raw muscle below a thick layer of oozing gray-green pus.

I wonder how I will be able to communicate with this extremely ill woman. Based on Ted's description, I expect to find her confused and incoherent. I am shocked when Carol's hazel eyes pop open and look into mine as she says, "I know you. You gave me that awful stuff that made me poop before you looked into my guts."

I quietly chuckle.

I notice her thoughts occasionally wander as she experiences hallucinatory voices coming from the empty bed next to her. Yet, Carol's mind is the clearest that it has been during this entire hospitalization.

I ask her several times, "Do you want to live?"

She responds, "I want to live. I have a lot to do. I don't want to die!" She understands that the surgeons will have to amputate both of her legs to save her life. Several times, she repeats, "I want them cut off. I don't care if I won't be able to walk again. Just don't let me die."

In my opinion, Carol meets the legal requirements of mental capacity at this moment. She is capable of choosing to live and to have the surgery.

J. Michael Gospe, M.D.

I ask her nurse to witness and confirm Carol's decisions and document them in the chart. Carol repeats what she previously said: "Have them cut off my legs, I want to live."

I breathe a sigh of relief. Her requests take priority over the wishes of her mother or daughter. I wish they could have heard Carol speak those words for themselves.

After I update Ted regarding Carol's verbal consent, he tells me he wants to hold off surgery as long as possible. He hopes her legs will show signs of healing on their own. Unfortunately, during the next few days her condition deteriorates. Ted schedules surgery without further delay.

On Friday morning, Carol enters the surgical department to await the start of her operation. While in my office seeing patients, I receive an emergency phone call from the Pre-Op nurse at the hospital. I hear Debra's angry voice yelling in the background, "Move my mother back to the ward!"

Sighing, the frustrated nurse pleads, "Doc, I need you right away, I can't do anything with that crazy woman. She insists that we take the patient back to her room. The chaplain is trying to calm her, but she won't listen to him. She is scaring the other patients."

I tell her, "I'll be right over."

As I walk-run into the Pre-Op Room, I find Debra arguing with the nurse and chaplain who are unable to insert a word between her rapid-fire vocalizations. She barely takes time to breathe between screams.

Carol, under sedation, is on a gurney. Her mother sits in a chair next to her, their fingers entwined. On the other side of the small room, two patients and their families also await surgery.

The noise in the Pre-Op Room shatters my thoughts. When I attempt to talk with the daughter in a calm voice, she turns away and continues her tirade. My mind flips between Carol's determination to live at all cost and Debra's determination to stop the surgery.

I know the right thing to do. I walk over to the nurse and softly say, "Wheel the patient into the O.R."

WE CAN, BUT SHOULD WE?

The nurse goes to the head of Carol's gurney, pushes it into the center of the room, swivels it ninety degrees, and moves Carol into the operating room corridor and the automatic doors close.

Much to my surprise, when Debra becomes aware of Carol's departure, she immediately calms down and goes to the waiting room to sit with her grandmother and the hospital chaplain.

Carol's surgery proceeds without difficulty. Following the operation, she improves both physically and mentally. Within twenty-four hours, she communicates with the staff in a lucid manner. Over the next few weeks, her psychiatrist adjusts her psychiatric medications. Carol is ready to work on accepting her new body image. Eventually, she is transferred from the hospital to a psychiatric rehabilitation unit where she continues intensive psychiatric therapy and is fitted with two prosthetic legs.

Seven years after Carol underwent surgery, her story still moves me. I want to include it in my memoir, *Learnings in an Elevator*. I write to her to ask for permission to use her story. Less than a week later, Carol sends me a short note penned in a beautiful script. She graciously gives me her approval to use this material as well as her authorization to contact her current psychiatrist.

Her psychiatrist informs me that he sees her twice a month. During the first few years after surgery, her emotional instability gradually eased. With the aid of several face-lifts and a change of hairstyle, she has created a new image for herself that matches her emotional wellness. There have been no further suicide attempts. He goes on to say that Carol has successfully discontinued the use of her tranquilizers. She enjoys a close relationship with Debra and two grandchildren, but has grown away from her mother. A new and improved set of prostheses is on the way. Carol hopes to learn to walk on her own for the first time since that fateful day so long ago

J. Michael Gospe, M.D.

Reflections
Non-maleficence

My professors at Stanford Medical School taught the meaning of the Latin phrase *primum non nocere* or *non-maleficence*, <u>first</u>, <u>do no harm</u>. The Hippocratic Oath implores a physician to:

> *...prescribe regimens for the good of my patients according to*
> *my ability and my judgment and never do harm to anyone.*

Every action we take in medicine should result in more benefit than burden for our patient. This seems self-evident. After all, why would anyone who entered a healing profession ever consider maiming his or her patient?

Carol's situation raised widely divergent viewpoints around the effects the amputations might have on her psyche. Would prolongation of her life lead to a fate worse than death? Her family was convinced that would be the case. The physicians were not sure.

A dilemma can develop when a physician in good conscience feels that his course of therapy will result in a definite benefit for his patient, whereas the patient or surrogate decision-maker may have an entirely different understanding. When there is a strong difference in opinion regarding the benefits or burdens of a specific treatment, the value of patient autonomy[1] trumps that of the physician and the family. Our patient, or her surrogate decision-maker, is the only one to determine if a treatment will result in a benefit for or a burden upon her. This can only happen after she receives and understands complete factual information about her options.

A strong similarity exists between the cases of Sally, the young girl in Chapter 2, *Changing Image,* and Carol. At the time I first met them, neither patient was able to voice her preferred treatment. In both scenarios physicians seriously considered major surgery to prolong life. The patients' loved ones declined surgery as they felt the burdens would outweigh the benefits of an operation. There was an important distinction between these two women. During her life, Sally could never speak for herself. Without the esophageal surgery, Sally's surgeons said she would experience recurrent lung infections, one of which would eventually take her life. Sally's father felt that having surgery and the withdrawal of her support systems would result in more suffering than he wished his daughter to undergo.

In contrast, Carol experienced a short but lucid time when she understood the significance of her condition. She spoke of her desire to live and to proceed with bilateral amputations of her legs. This contrasted with the fearful projections made by her family who had seen her battle severe depression leading up to multiple suicide attempts. They were certain that the loss of both of her legs would result in a life *not worth living*. Meanwhile, her physicians told the family that without surgery, Carol would face an agonizing death with severe pain in her legs, putrefying flesh, and uncontrollable sepsis.

I am grateful Carol regained her capacity long enough to express her wishes and give me the authority to act in her behalf.

Experience teaches me to honor the complexity of the various voices surrounding a dilemma. Sally and Carol's stories both had unexpected endings. Sally flourished without surgery, living her life in the company of those who love her. Carol rose to the challenge of a new life.

We must never ignore the resilience of the human spirit.

---

1.   Chapter 1: *Living Life on the Edge* (Autonomy)

4
The Shadow Side
Justice

Dorothy Greenfield has been on the oncology ward for an extended stay. The staff feels that they cannot give her adequate care because of constant pressure exerted by her overbearing partner, Ms. Chapman who insists on monitoring every procedure. She is present day and night.

A soft voice spoke when I picked up the phone. "Is Dr. Gospe there?"

"Speaking."

"I'm Susan Carter, the new nurse manager for 1 Central East. I have an ethical issue I'd like to discuss with you. Is this a good time?"

"Sure. What do you have Susan?"

"My staff is having control issues with a patient's partner. She intervenes whenever they begin to administer necessary skilled nursing care."

I reach for a pen and pad of paper by the phone. "Tell me a bit about the patient."

"Dorothy Greenfield, age fifty-three, came to the hospital four months ago with a bowel obstruction. The surgeons removed a blockage caused by a widespread and aggressive endometrial carcinoma. They were forced to take out all but three and one-half feet of her small bowel. The oncologist feels we have done all we can for her in the hospital. He recommends switching her from active treatment to comfort care in a skilled nursing facility."

26

WE CAN, BUT SHOULD WE?

"Why has she been in the hospital so long?"

Susan sighs. "Ms. Greenfield needs intravenous hyperalimentation feedings because her short gut cannot absorb oral nutrition."

"What's the ethical issue?"

Susan pauses. "The big problem is Ms. Chapman, her partner. Over time she has gradually increased her presence in the patient's room. Now, she is there twenty-four/seven. She insists that she is the only one who can turn Ms. Greenfield in bed and to clean her surgical wounds. She records all visits and all medications and treatments in a notebook, including the names and titles of medical personnel. Her distrusting attitude intimidates the staff and creates a barrier between the patient and her assigned caregivers.

In addition, both the patient and her partner demand to be seen by an alternative medical care practitioner. They will not accept the fact such practitioners are not on our staff. The truth is Ms. Greenfield is actively dying from the cancer. There is no further medical therapy to change her outcome."

"How is the staff handling this?"

Susan lowers her voice. "They are reluctant to be assigned to her care. Every time one of the nurses moves to change a dressing, adjust IV fluids, or examine Ms. Greenfield, Ms. Chapman interrupts. They feel frustrated because they are not allowed to practice the prescribed standard of nursing care." Susan swallows and clears her throat. "They worry that Ms. Greenfield will develop skin ulcers and sepsis because of the lack of proper attention."

"Does Ms. Greenfield have capacity? What does she say about this?"

"It is impossible to have a private conversation with her because of Ms. Chapman's interference. She seems pretty clear to me. At the same time, she allows Ms. Chapman to speak for her."

I can feel tension arising in me as I listen to this untenable situation. "Is there any way to reason with them?"

"At this point, no. We barely communicate. The staff is at an impasse to break through Ms. Chapman's power. Everyone's afraid they might be sued if they push her too far."

I take a deep breath. "I'll be over this afternoon to visit with them."

J. Michael Gospe, M.D.

When I speak with the nurses caring for Ms. Greenfield, I can't help but notice their irritation and anger. They confirm Susan's summation of the smoldering climate between the women and the staff.

I walk into the patient's room and meet unexpected disarray. Papers and books are piled on the windowsill. A recliner chair stands in the corner with a blanket strewn over its back and onto the floor. An emaciated lady lies in the bed, covers askew. She looks up at me with dull eyes.

I introduce myself. Before she can respond, a tall middle-aged woman, I assume to be Ms. Chapman, steps out from the nearby bathroom. With a strong authoritative voice and no introduction, she demands, "Who are you? Give me your card!"

I'm not prepared for the intensity of her interrogation. I collect myself and apologize, "I'm sorry. I'm Dr. Gospe, from the ethics department."

"Then sign your legal name on this piece of paper." She pushes a pad of lined paper in front of my face. Today's date heads the top of the page, but it is otherwise empty.

When I begin the interview, I make it a point to direct my questions to Ms. Greenfield. As Ms. Chapman answers each one, I imagine Ms. Greenfield's presence shrink before my eyes. Within seconds, I feel suffocated and leave the room.

Susan nods as I describe my experience. She tells me, "The staff is stymied as to how to alter the situation."

After a moment, I ask "Isn't it against hospital policy to let visitors spend the night here, much less allow them to perform nursing procedures on patients?"

"Yes. Truthfully, the nurses were pleased to have Ms. Chapman's presence at first. She assisted with some basic help like massaging her friend's back and legs and kept her company. Before we knew it, she took on the direction of her care, telling the nurses what to do. Then she moved on to staying the night."

Susan continues, "We realize Ms. Greenfield depends on her friend to be her intermediary. Under these circumstances, we feel strongly that forcing Ms. Chapman to leave after visiting hours would adversely affect Ms. Greenfield's emotional state."

WE CAN, BUT SHOULD WE?

Susan adds, "We get little support from the doctors. They have brief contact during hospital rounds. They are in and out in a flash. Our frustration must seem unfounded to them, though it's hard for me to believe they are oblivious to the room's caustic atmosphere."

I take some time to organize my thoughts. A conference with the staff to discuss our various findings and any options is crucial. We must come to a plan of action before the oncologist and primary nurse present any recommendations.

At the meeting, we explore a bit of the history of these two women. They have lived nearly half their lives together. Over the years, they have developed a close bond that has resulted in one of them significantly being dominant and overprotective and the other being passively dependent. Our focus is to work within the confines of their unique relationship. We also admit we cannot undo what has evolved over the last four months.

When the oncologist and nurse meet with the two women, they explain once again that medical therapy and further acute hospitalization are no longer helpful for Ms. Greenfield. They acknowledge the women's wish for alternative therapy and repeat the fact that there are no alternative medical practitioners on the hospital staff. The only way they can obtain this type of consultation is to move to an outpatient setting. All agree that the location of the women's residence is too remote from medical, nursing, and hospice services.

The women continue to refuse a transfer to a skilled nursing facility unless Ms. Chapman would be able to stay the night. They do agree to think about other options. In the meantime, the staff's anger and frustration remains unabated.

It takes another month of hospitalization before Ms. Greenfield and Ms. Chapman will consider a long-term hotel with a hospital bed. Support from hospice and an alternative medical practitioner would also be possible in this setting.

Our social worker finds a spacious hotel room in another county. Two days after her transfer, Ms. Greenfield becomes unresponsive. The last information we have is that she is taken by ambulance to a nearby hospital where she is admitted to the ICU.

Nine months later, I was surprised to receive a Christmas card from Ms. Chapman. She thanked me for *standing there even if it was mostly in the shadows.* She said that Ms. Greenfield expired almost immediately after entering the hospital. I responded with a note of sympathy. She replied with a long and sensitive letter containing information about Ms. Greenfield past, including several photographs.

She writes a human-interest story about a vibrant Ms. Greenfield. Dorothy had been a television director, an Emmy winning producer for a public television documentary, a composer of six original music albums, and a writer of two screenplays and a book of poetry.

I am struck by the contrast of my shrunken image of Ms. Greenfield as she lay in her disheveled bed and the description of her younger self that Ms. Chapman shares with me. Even today, I feel the loss in knowing only a slim shadow of Dorothy's life while she was in our care.

Reflections

Justice

The value of justice encompasses fairness and equity. It invites us to welcome the stranger in our midst who has a story to tell, a story that reveals a depth beyond the hospital bed and room number. Often, these stories lay buried by the stresses of our patient's illness and the strangeness of the hospital setting. It is for a caregiver to have a mistaken first impression of his patient. The truth is there is always more than one's eye or intuition can see.

Physicians and nurses desire to do everything they can for their sick patients. Frustration and burnout are common because of the demands of any given day upon the staff. Two conditions that can impair the quality of medical care include the seriousness of the staff's patient load and the upheaval of routines when communication breaks down between staff, patients, and families. At the same time, patients and families want to be assured their loved one is receiving the best of care. They want the staff to hear them, to respect them, and to comfort them.

WE CAN, BUT SHOULD WE?

When Alice Chapman embedded herself into Dorothy Greenfield's care, the nurses lose their ability to be objective and empathetic. They lost sight of their patient as an individual by choosing to limit their contact within this dysfunction. This resulted in less than ideal care and support for both Ms. Greenfield and Ms. Chapman as they found themselves covered with a patina of discontent.

Our team, including myself, failed to see Dorothy Greenfield as a person when we focused on Ms. Chapman as *the problem*. If we had only considered Ms. Chapman as the *stranger in the midst*, one with complete access to our patient's story. Instead, we strove to isolate one from the other. We missed the chance to develop a gateway toward a working relationship based on the long history these two women shared.

Ms. Chapman was watching her dear friend dying. What was she feeling: guilt, grief, anxiety, or utter exhaustion? I wonder what difference it would have made if I asked Ms. Chapman, *"How are you?"* or *"What would you like me to know about Dorothy?"* If only I could have risen above what I judged to be an untenable situation and instead just focused on our patient and surrogate together, as allies seeking a common goal.

The learning here is for the professional instead to take *time out* to tease apart the issues at hand. To look at a situation with an open mind and without blame helps generate creative ways that have been hidden in the mire of emotions. Most of all, it is imperative to not take the patient or their family's behavior personally. Rather, it is up to the professional staff to note the stress the patient and surrogate are experiencing. It is not uncommon for a patient and family to feel they have lost their identity while they are at the mercy of the hospital's foreign culture. Yet, they must make end of life decisions while feeling fearful and anxious about the dying process and the immanent loss of a loved one. The patient and family need the medical team's support. As professionals, we must admit we can become immune to a patient's and family's quandary as they live through saying goodbye. We can help by simply checking in with a soft voice and a light touch. "How are you feeling today?"

31

J. Michael Gospe, M.D.

In this time of endings, the patient's spirituality or religion can offer the salve of healing, where the medical reality cannot. It is my view that dying invites all of us to surrender to the moment of *what is*. How we incorporate our spiritual self in the process is for each one of us to discover. A pastor, counselor, hospital chaplain, or hospice worker can be invaluable at these times.

Here are some questions I ask myself when I feel uncomfortable with a patient:

- *What do I know about this person's life, his family?*
- *What keeps me from accepting my patient and family as they are?*

As a healthcare professional, when you find yourself taking care of a patient who makes you uncomfortable or as a family member feeling alienated by the medical staff, ask yourself: *Am I getting lost in a problem? Am I reacting from a place within me that has nothing to do with the situation at hand?*

When we step back, new information may come forward to clear the air and place a totally new light and energy on the situation, allowing everyone to work more effectively together.

These following questions are beneficial for patient, family, and staff:

- *How could I have recognized the developing dilemma sooner?*
- *Did I bring my concerns about potential jeopardy of patient care to the nursing manager early enough to nip harm to the patient?*
- *Have I switched my demeanor from compassion to anger or even indifference or avoidance?*
- *Do I feel devalued and unappreciated?*
- *If so, am I aware of the reason for the frustrations that arise in me?*
- *Was I aware that consultation with the bioethics department as a team of professionals could help clarify the issues at hand?*
- *Did I remember the dying process is a spiritual one?*

WE CAN, BUT SHOULD WE?

The members of the medical team and family care about our patient. We want to give of our best selves. We all want to relieve pain and suffering and offer a healing touch in the midst of the worst of times. When we do, we are acting with justice and with equity.

5
The Small Card
Fidelity

Penny Worthington, a forty-five year-old woman, presented to the Emergency Room at the county hospital with an upper gastrointestinal bleed due to esophogeal varicies. When the doctors diagnosed the bleeding to be life threatening, they advised a blood transfusion. At that point, her husband presented them with two printed cards: both identified Penny as a Jehovah Witness who did not want a blood transfusion under any circumstances.

It is just after midnight when the shrill ring of my bedside telephone jars me from a deep slumber. I feel the normal rush of adrenaline rush of an on call night as my mind struggles toward some degree of alertness.

I hear, "Dr. Gospe, I have Dr. Neville holding for you."

I recognize the voice on the line. It is the night operator for my answering service. Sometimes I wonder how she puts up with the confused voices of sleepy doctors. "Put him on, Flo."

Bruce Neville is a second-year primary care resident at Sonoma County Hospital where I am one of the mentor-consultants to young medical residents at the County Hospital. I round with them on their hospitalized patients and am available to them when they face difficult gastrointestinal problems.

"Mike." Bruce begins. "Sorry to wake you, but you're on GI call tonight, aren't you?"

WE CAN, BUT SHOULD WE?

With my voice still somewhat groggy, I answer, "Mmmmm. What do you have?"

"We've got an upper GI bleeder in the E.R. She's a 45 year-old chronic alcoholic who is pouring a mixture of bright red blood and coffee grounds out of her mouth. Her vitals stink. She has a BP of 80 over 50 with a pulse of 135. Her hemoglobin is 8.5 and dropping. I wanted to start blood, but her husband gave me two cards that say she's a Jehovah Witness and refuses blood products. I'm filling her with Ringers Lactate but I'm afraid that won't help her vitals if she doesn't stop bleeding soon. I need your help."

I quickly play a well-rehearsed scenario in my mind: lavage the stomach of clot, pass a scope, coagulate, or sclerose the bleeding site, and keep my fingers crossed. "Wake up the Endo Team and have them bring the gastroscope to the ER. I'll be there in 10 minutes." I hang up the phone and dress. On my way to the car, I reach into the cookie jar for a chocolate chip cookie, my habitual reward in the night.

I meet Bruce in the ER and quickly examine his patient, Mrs. Penny Worthington. A large bore nasal-gastric tube drains copious amounts of clotted old and new blood from her stomach. Her vital signs are as advertised. The endoscopy nurse arrives with the scope as I complete my evaluation and obtain an urgent consent for the procedure from Mr. Worthington. Within five minutes we have the equipment ready and proceed with the gastroscopy.

Although visualization is poor because of the rapid bleeding, I am able to locate the source of her blood loss. She has a giant esophageal variceal vein with a fresh clot adherent to its surface. I stop the bleeding by injecting a sclerosing agent into the vessel. The whole procedure takes less than ten minutes. For the moment, the bleeding has stopped. Afterwards, I update Mr. Worthington with my findings.

He is a large man in his fifties. He sits with his wife's mother and father in a row of chairs in the hallway. I tell the three of them my findings. Mr. Worthington admits that his wife is a chronic alcoholic. This is no surprise to me in view of the hard knobby liver I feel in her abdomen and the huge blood vessels I see in her esophagus. I tell him we will comply with his wife's wishes not to have a blood transfusion.

Mr. Worthington, no longer a quiet and concerned listener, glares at me. In a gruff loud voice, he says, "I want her to receive blood."

I note to myself an abrupt change: *Mr. Worthington presented the cards yet he does not want to honor them.* I look at the three in family members in front of me. "Did Mrs. Worthington ever discuss the issue of blood transfusions with any of you?"

"No."

Her parents do not admit to knowing Penny's denial regarding blood transfusions. I look at the two cards. They both identified her as a Jehovah Witness. Both clearly state she does not want blood products administrated. Both carry her signature. One card bears a date twelve years ago. Neither card was witnessed. My question is, *Do these cards speak for her today?*

Mr. Worthington threatens, "I'm going to sue the hospital and doctors if my wife doesn't receive blood that she needs to live."

"Sir, I must follow your wife's wishes. In this case, they legally overpower what you and her parents want done."

Mrs. Worthington is stable after the scoping and Bruce and I arrange to transfer her to the ICU. By this time she is in a deep coma because of liver failure and an accumulation of ammonia produced by the digestion of the blood in her intestinal tract.

I fill Bruce in with my discussion with Mr. Worthington. He reasons, "Since she is a chronic alcoholic, there is no way she could be a practicing Jehovah Witness. I think that her life style negates those cards and she should have blood. Besides, she will bleed to death without the transfusion."

I take an alternate view, "Look, Bruce. It doesn't matter if she drinks or not. Our patient carried at least one of those cards for twelve years. She has had ample opportunity to remove them from her purse if she changed her mind. I feel we must honor her wishes. Anything else would be unethical and, from a legal basis, would be battery."

I return home shortly after three in the morning. I slip into bed after treating myself to another chocolate chip cookie. Less than fifteen minutes later I am beginning to relax and doze off when Bruce calls with an update.

WE CAN, BUT SHOULD WE?

"Mike, she seems relatively stable, but her husband is ranting and raving about suing the pants off of everyone if we don't give her blood. Her hemoglobin is floating around eight grams. The nurses and I are uneasy about doing nothing. The guy scares us with his threats. Can we please give her a unit or two?"

I am sleepy and uncomfortable with the situation concerning Mrs. Worthington's status. I had been on the Ethics Committee for a bit over a year and am reasonably certain that her Jehovah Witness Cards trump her family's wishes. However, I cannot ignore Bruce and the nurses' angst as they face her husband's anger. I reluctantly agree to Bruce giving his patient two units of whole blood. Yet, my mind is unsettled as I replay the events of the evening.

Two days later, Mrs. Worthington's coma lightens and she regains consciousness. I still feel troubled about authorizing the transfusions in the first place and am compelled to inform her about them. In my opinion, not doing so would create a major severing of trust between her and the medical profession. I tell my colleagues of my intention. Much to my distress, several of the other physicians on the case strongly disagree. Nevertheless, I am adamant.

I am in a somber mood when I enter her room and sit down next to her bed. I empathize with Mr. Worthington's desire to save his wife's life at all costs, even to the point of denying her personal wishes. I feel it best not to reveal her husband's emotional distress in the decision-making process.

After examining her and checking on her current complaints, I look into her eyes and say, "Penny. The bleeding was heavy. Since your Jehovah Witness cards were not witnessed, there was concern about their validity. We felt it necessary to give you a blood transfusion the night that you came to the hospital."

She was silent for a few moments and then responded, "I hear you, Doc. But, in the future, I don't want to receive blood products even if my life is at risk." She then adds, "I understand why blood was given to me and I'm not angry."

I touch her hand, "Please make your wishes clearly known to your husband and family. When you feel better, update a new card and

J. Michael Gospe, M.D.

sign it. Make certain it is witnessed. This will assure your wishes will be followed."

Reflections
Fidelity

Fidelity is the value of being faithful[1] or loyal in our dealings with patients. The professional staff wants to honor their patient's wishes. In order to do that, we need a foundation upon which to base appropriate treatment plans. Ideally, we look to the capable[2] patient for direction. It is more difficult if he does not have capacity. In that situation, we need to discover if he had previously filled out a legal document containing his wishes. This could be an Advance Health Care Document (AHCD)[3], Physician Order for Life-Sustaining Treatment (POLST), or, as with Mrs. Worthington, a Jehovah Witness Card. It is most important he discuss his values with a legally appointed surrogate[4], a close relative, a friend, or a staff member.

Fidelity in medicine is more than just telling the truth; it is accepting the beliefs and behaviors of the patient. This is especially true when those of the family, staff, and institution differ from that of the patient. When well-meaning people force their own issues and desires into the treatment options, they can *override* those of the patient.

The physician has a responsibility to balance what the patient wants done with what is medically, legally, and ethically appropriate. The doctor must explain the reasoning behind the offered therapy in a truthful and direct manner and in a way that the patient and family can understand.

I met Mrs. Worthington in the 1980's, early in my exposure to medical ethics. Then, the standard of medical care was to transfuse a patient if her hemoglobin was below 10 grams. There was a great deal of anxiety among members of the medical community regarding withholding of the transfusion of blood products to Jehovah Witnesses when their hemoglobin dropped below the acceptable levels to sustain life. It was not uncommon for a physician to transfuse units of blood secretly, often against a patient's expressed wishes.

38

WE CAN, BUT SHOULD WE?

When we attempted to honor Mrs. Worthington's desires concerning blood transfusions, we faced several difficulties. Although her two cards gave us a strong indication of what she wanted, her family brought confusion into the mix when they denied knowledge of her intent. Mr. Worthington, who presented the cards to Dr. Neville, clearly placed his personal wishes over those of his wife when faced with the possibility of her immanent death. A crisis ensued when he demanded that the staff proceed with transfusions or he would proceed to file a lawsuit. The fact that the norm of practice was to give blood to sustain life, even against a patient's wishes, muddied the waters even more.

Once Mrs. Worthington regained capacity, I felt responsible to tell her what happened when she was in crisis. I understood that keeping the secret would coerce both family and staff to lie. Eventually, the secret would surface through her medical records.

Not to inform the patient of her diagnosis, treatment, or prognosis is a form of deceit by all involved: family and professionals. These secrets may well promote distrust and undermine the last wishes of the patient who may become isolated from intimate and much needed support.

In a situation where the family insists on not telling their elderly grandmother she has terminal cancer, they are forced to create false explanations for her pain and weight loss. When further evidence of the body shutting down occurs, the stories no longer hold. To keep *the secret* masks the integrity of all professionals and family alike. In truth, it is most likely that the patient knows the seriousness of her diagnosis. Were she accidently to hear the truth from whispered comments, she would question the veracity of those whom she has put her trust when she is most dependent and vulnerable. As my father, an OB/GYN physician once told me, "When you tell the truth, you do not have to question what you said."

On the other hand, a distressed patient may choose not[5] to be informed regarding *the bad news* of her declining status. Then, she must choose an individual to receive and convey this information to loved ones.

Another patient may say, "Don't tell my family that I know I am dying. They don't think I understand what is going on and they don't want me to worry." It is best to gently suggest to the patient that she does not have to protect her family from her knowing the truth. Once the family is relieved from the deception, they may openly grieve together and comfort their loved one in her last days.

I have found that care conferences[6] are invaluable in pooling the expertise of doctors, nurses, and spiritual counselors with the questions and concerns of patient and family. The review of current medical findings and options for further care opens discussion that often leads to understanding by all and can be a vehicle of comfort and support during a most difficult time.

Changes in medical and societal thought have occurred during the past few decade regarding the concept of patient self-determination. The courts have repeatedly upheld the understanding that patients with capacity, or their surrogates, have the right to accept or refuse any form of medical care if the burdens of the treatment outweigh the benefits from the *patient's*[7] point of view. For the medical community to do otherwise is considered a form of battery, unless the courts order that therapy.

With respect to this case, many Jehovah Witnesses believe that their acceptance of blood will affect their ability to obtain eternal life. An adult Witness who feels this way generally documents this information by means of a Jehovah Witness medical directive card that has been signed, dated, and witnessed. It clearly states the signer's refusal of treatment that involves blood products. Once hospital personnel become aware of this fact, they have an ethical and legal obligation to follow these wishes.

When we gave blood to Mrs. Worthington, the value of fidelity *demanded* that we inform her what was done to her body at a time when she did not have the capacity to speak for herself. Although I didn't think of it when I spoke to her, I now wish I had suggested to her and her family to invite a Jehovah Witness minister to be present during this crisis.

Where life and death issues are involved, we, as caregivers, must remember that a patient's spirituality awakens during the dying process. It could supersede the direction of medical treatment.

WE CAN, BUT SHOULD WE?

1.   Chapter 17: *Further Reflections* (Dignity)
2.   Chapter 7: *Window of Opportunity* (Capacity)
3.   Chapter 9: *"Listen to Me!"* (Advance Health Care Directive)
4.   Chapter 8: *Whose on First* (Surrogacy)
5.   Chapter 10: *No Man is an Island* (Communication)
6.   Chapter 11: *"I Love My Son"* (Case Conferences)
7.   Chapter 1: *Living Life on the Edge* (Autonomy)

6
Kitty Cats
Goals of Therapy

Gertrude Frederick is seventy-four, without friends or family. She has severe kidney disease. Surgery may improve her condition, but only temporarily. Mrs. Frederick lacks consistent capacity. She does not have a surrogate decision-maker. She is firm about wanting to return home to her cats. Her urologist requests an ethics consultation to help determine Mrs. Fredrick's appropriate treatment.

The phone interrupts my concentration. I glance at the phone's Caller ID and see *Schneider, F*, a name from out of my past. Frank is a urologist. I put a mark in my book and pick up the phone. "Hello?"

I recognize Frank's distinctive deep voice at once. "Is Doctor Gospe available?"

"Hi, Frank. This is Mike. What can I do for you?"

"You're still involved in ethics, aren't you?"

"Yes," I answer, "How have you been? It's been a long time since I've spoken to you. What's cooking?"

"I'm between a rock and a hard place. I have this pleasantly demented elderly lady in the hospital. I'm pretty sure surgery can extend her life. I've visited with her on a number of occasions and showed her diagrams about what is happening to her kidneys. She won't listen to me. She wants to get home to her cats. Period." Frank sighed, "Mike, I know she doesn't understand the seriousness of her condition, much less her options at this point. I'm unable to find a way to explain the facts so she can understand them."

"Is there any family or friend you can speak with?"

"Her husband used to take care of her, but he died a number of years ago. Her only relative is a nephew who lives over a hundred miles away. She burned all of her bridges with him as well as with her neighbors. Her nephew refuses to take part in making any medical decisions for her. The poor lady is all alone except for her three cats."

With paper and pencil at hand, I ask, "What's her medical problem?"

"She has retroperitoneal fibrosis complicated with extensive renal calcification. Solid masses of stone fill the pelvis of her left kidney and most of her bladder. Also, a fibrous stricture of her right ureter is compromising that kidney. The only thing that might help her would be to remove her left kidney, open up her bladder to attempt to remove the massive calcium deposits embedded in it, and place a stent in the right ureter to allow drainage of her remaining kidney."

"What do you think would be best for her?"

Frank sighs. "I just don't know." He pauses for a moment and continues. "If I operate, she should move into a long term facility to receive skilled nursing care and to be assured of keeping her doctor's appointments. But," Frank lets out a deep breath, "she clearly doesn't want to do that. Like I said before, all she wants to do is to return home and be with those darn cats." He adds, "If she does that, she'll die of renal failure in a matter of months."

I think for a second and look up at him. "Your goals of therapy are to minimize her suffering. Her goals are to continue her life living alone with her cats. The problem boils down to either prolonging her life with complicated and extensive surgery, long-term rehabilitation, and close medical follow-up or sending her back home with her cats where she will have to fend for herself and die of renal failure or sepsis within a short time. From what you are saying, she longs to be in familiar surroundings with her cats, her only friends. She can't imagine being anywhere else. In either scenario she will need caregivers. I wonder how she might adapt to strangers in her home. We both know that to send her home alone with her cats is not a viable option."

I look at my notes. "Let's call a case conference with the staff. The key here is to provide a broad spectrum of ideas for her care from as many of the physicians and staff involved in her case as possible. We can put our heads together and, hopefully, come up with a plan that that includes tending to her medical needs in a way that helps meet her goals."

I drop by the surgical floor to meet Mrs. Frederick. I am most interested to learn how she perceives her future beyond her need to care for her cats. *What does she understand?*

I walk into her room where I see a quiet lady lying askew in bed with a bit of a vacant stare in her eyes. The bed sheets cover only a small portion of her thin frame. Pasty skin hangs from her face and body, a mark of recent extensive weight loss. Mrs. Frederick is drowsy. She looks up at me.

"Hello, Mrs. Fredrick. I'm Dr. Gospe. Dr. Schneider asked me to meet you. Do you know where you are?"

"I'm in a hospital. They tell me that something isn't working when I make my water, but nothing hurts. I don't know why they won't let me go back home. I want to go home. My kitties need me. I miss them."

She smiles when tell her, "Don't' worry, your cats are well cared for. One of your neighbors took them to the vet after you entered the hospital last week."

It becomes clear to me that she does not understand her medical status and does not have the capacity to process her frail condition and the resulting nursing and medical needs it imposes.

After my visit, I review that day's notes in the medical record and find that Mrs. Frederick is eating well, voiding on her own, and physically able to get out of bed without help. Because of her confusion, her nurses advise twenty-four hour assistance if she were to return to live at home.

With a list in hand, I personally invite each of her doctors to a conference for the next afternoon. I ask Sally, our social worker, to contact her manager. She will also invite the head nurse in the ICU and a representative from the Adult Protective Services (APS). I contact legal representation from the hospital's administration to complete a broad circle of information and support.

WE CAN, BUT SHOULD WE?

The turnout for the care conference includes five physicians: her family doctor for many years, the hospitalist, chief of the palliative care team, chief medical officer of the hospital, Frank, and me. We also have Sally, her manager, the floor's head nurse, and a representative of APS.

I welcome the group and update everyone with Mrs. Frederick's current medical situation and paint the picture of the dilemma. "Surgery would be extremely complex and would require her to have close medical follow-up care by both her internist and urologist." I continue, "Mrs. Fredrick has repeatedly told a number of people that she does not want to leave her cats because they need her. She doesn't want surgery. However," I add, "based on their direct examination of the patient, all of her physicians agree: she does not have the capacity to make her own medical decisions. Nor can she care for herself at home. What we don't know is how she would adapt to twenty-four hour in-home care?"

My eyes focus on Frank. I then look around the room to see a group of professionals, each with many years of experience in their field. Their contact with Mrs. Frederick varies from hours to decades and they are prepared to do what they can to help her. "The questions are: *Do we force an operation on her and send her to a skilled nursing facility against her wishes? What has to be in place before we can allow this confused patient to go home to her cats to die of renal failure or sepsis?*"

We have a productive hour with everyone able to share his or her thoughts. Her family doctor fills us in on his experiences with Mrs. Fredrick. "Although her capacity seems to ebb and flow over the years, she is slowly getting worse even with adjustments of her medications. She has a terrible history of keeping appointments with me; she misses more than she keeps." He groans a bit as he continues, "All she seems to care about are her three cats. She rambles on and on about them as she avoids hearing facts regarding her medical condition. I sent her to Frank three years ago to evaluate her kidney problem."

Frank sighs deeply as he chimes in, "I recommended surgery several times since I first saw Mrs. Frederick. She always refused my suggestions. If I operate, I would need to see her frequently to treat

45

early infections and I know I'd have to replace the stent periodically as continuing fibroses will compromise it. In my opinion, her body will have no chance at all to heal if she doesn't get follow up care. I really don't want to operate on a patient who won't keep appointments to see me in my office. Its too darn dangerous." He adds, "In her case, doing nothing will result in renal failure and death, probably within months."

Sally glances at her notes as she points out, "Not only did Mrs. Fredrick frequently fail many of her appointments with her physicians, she also won't let home nursing services or APS into her house. I spoke with her nephew who has helped her with her finances in the past, but he hasn't seen her for several years and doesn't want to get involved."

The APS worker, obviously frustrated, unconsciously twirls a lock of hair as she speaks up. "Mrs. Frederick tied our hands by consistently refusing any and all assistance that we have offered to help her coordinate community resources so she can live independently and safely."

Further discussion leads us to agree: an operation is not a viable option. We would like to honor Mrs. Frederick's goal of going home to her cats. We do agree that it is inappropriate to discharge her on her own without a safety net in place. Sally will work on establishing home care and follow-up for the patient. Her family doctor will continue to make appointments with her, but is not hopeful that she will keep them. The APS worker will reopen the file for Mrs. Fredrick and work with the home care personnel.

Mrs. Frederick goes home two days after the meeting. We make arrangements for a community case manager, Irene, to make a home visit and find a caregiver to help. Upon arriving at the home, Irene discovers that Mrs. Frederick's dementia is far worse than the hospital imagined. Fleas, filth, feces, and urine saturate the house. The cats' litter box looks as if she hadn't changed it in over a year. Irene calls 911. The emergency responders agree that it isn't safe to have her in the house and they take her to the emergency room.

Mrs. Frederick reenters the hospital. With a great deal of urging, she agrees to go into a care home. Sally contacts Mrs. Frederick's nephew again. This time, he agrees to become his aunt's legal conservator. Her dementia rapidly advances. Before long, she forgets about her cats that are now living in an animal shelter. As expected, her renal failure gradually advances. She dies peacefully eight months later. Although she does not meet her goal of spending the rest of her life at home with her cats, her last months in her confused world are peaceful and comfortable.

Reflections
Goals of Therapy

We all have unique life goals that depend on an infinite number of factors that touch each of us throughout our life. When you imagine yourself at the end of your life are you one to say *I'm tired--please let me go,* or *I'm not ready yet--what are my options,* or *I have too much to live for—do everything.* Often we ignore these thoughts. They raise our defenses. We don't want to face the inevitable of suffering, losing control, or surrendering our will to the dying process.

When walking on the road toward our loved one or patient's death, we need to know their desires when medical choices are available. We need to ask her what she wants us to do when she has the capacity to make her own decisions. Formulating these goals is not easy. Not only do they depend upon the fabric of one's life, but also they often change over time as the medical condition evolves and different options present themselves. Ongoing communication is essential.

Mrs. Frederick was clear in her request. She never wavered over the course of her hospitalization. She let all of us know that she needed her kitties and they needed her!

There are circumstances when wishes cannot be honored as with Mrs. Frederick. Her failing mental condition and her unclean and unsafe home did not allow her to live alone with her beloved felines. She did not have any legal papers expressing her wishes. To make matters worse, she had no friends and the only relative our social worker could find was a reluctant nephew who, at first, would not agree to step in for his aunt.

47

Even though she lacked capacity, the hospital staff and I wanted to honor Mrs. Frederick's long-term goals until we realized it was not safe to do so. The California Probate Code[1] makes it clear that a physician or hospital is *not required to provide health care contrary to generally accepted health care standards* and *can decline a request for reasons of conscience.* Consequently, it was up to us to develop a plan that was both safe and appropriate. Needing to think creatively, we brought together a *community of concern* to participate in a case conference and establish a treatment plan for her.

It is important for all of us, whether we are healthcare workers or lay people, to consider how we want to spend the rest of our life and to share our thoughts verbally and in writing with our physician and loved ones. It is important for both family members and medical personnel to avoid superimposing their own individual preferences on their loved one or the patient. They must ask themselves, *what are the desires of our wife, husband, mom, dad, and patient?*

One's end of life goals may vary from:

- *I don't want to die. Do everything you can to keep me alive.*
- *I want to be alert to the end. Let me be with my family, hold their hands, and kiss their cheeks.*
- *I want to be pain free even if that means you have to put me into a deep sleep as my death approaches.*
- *Let me end it all now. Give me a magic drug that will send me to instant oblivion.*

It is our duty to our patient to keep an open mind and to do the best we can in the present moment with whatever evidence is available to us.

---

1.   Cal. Prob. Code § 4734

7
Window of Opportunity
Capacity

Charlie Phillips is a sixty-four year-old homeless man who lacks the capacity to make his own decisions. He severed contact with his family years ago and has no known friends. Mr. Phillips experienced a severe head injury after an automobile struck him. He remains unresponsive and is receiving life-support. His physician requests an ethics evaluation to help determine further treatment.

It is a rainy Saturday morning in early December. I just completed an urgent ethics case conference and was dictating my thoughts on one of the ICU computers. I saw Fred Wright looking in my direction.

Fred is the hospital's newest neurosurgeon. I met him six months ago at one of my monthly ethics seminars for new staff physicians where I wet the doctors' appetite regarding help we offer with medial ethical decisions. Since then, I have assisted Fred on several occasions.

"Mike. Do you have a sec? I'd like to share some thoughts with you about one of my patients."

I nod and I put the final touches on my consultation note. I look at Fred. His worried brow speaks volumes of unease.

"Mr. Phillips is unconscious. The social worker has spent the past couple of days trying to locate family or friends to help us make decisions for him." He adds, "I know what I would want done for me if I were the patient, but I don't have any idea what he'd want us to do for him."

J. Michael Gospe, M.D.

"Start at the beginning; bring me up to date. Sometimes important clues appear in telling the story."

"Two nights ago, he tried to cross Fourth Street after midnight. A hit and run car going fifty-five whopped him. When he arrived at the ER, he was unresponsive. An emergency MRI revealed blood on his brain. I performed an urgent craniotomy that night." Fred shakes his head. "The police told the ambulance crew that he lived under one of the bridges over the creek. None of the other squatters admitted to the police that they knew anything about him or the accident. My guess is that they were afraid of what might happen if they gave the authorities any information."

Fred pauses as he pulls his right ear lobe. "It's pretty clear to me that my patient isn't going to make it out of the hospital alive. I want to switch my goal of treatment for him to comfort care, but don't know if its legal for me to do that."

I look into Room 246 where Mr. Phillips lay covered by a single sheet. I see a cachectic elderly man with a battered body. Wires from him lead to computer screens to record the ups and downs of his vital signs. Fresh dressings hide his skull and most of his face from view. Several plastic bags containing blood and medications hang from two IV poles. A noisy mechanical respirator with its constant to-an-fro sigh brings oxygen into his lungs. A catheter drains urine from his bladder into a bag attached to the frame of his bed.

It is clear to me that Mr. Phillips lacks any reserves to fight his many injuries. And most important, he is alone, without friends, without a voice.

Fred groans and takes a breath, frustrated. "His blood alcohol level was sky high at 0.38 percent. These alcoholics really get me down. I get one or two of them a week with various types of head trauma. I work my butt off to repair their neurological damage. If they get out of the hospital, they return with other complications from alcohol, over and over and over and over again."

I nod my head at an all too common story. I agree with Fred as I reflect on my thirty years as a gastroenterologist. I had my share of alcoholic patients with liver disease, upper GI bleeding, pancreatitis, and a myriad of other conditions directly related to the abuse of alcohol. The majority of my patients found it impossible to

50

permanently abstain from drinking. Thus, the progressive destruction of their organs continued and often caused death. I, too, felt hopeless in motivating them towards a healthier lifestyle for their body and for their psyches.

Fred looks at Mr. Phillips' Electronic Medical Record (EMR) on the screen in front of him. "In the last month alone, he has had two admissions for alcoholic pancreatitis followed by three trips to the ER with acute intoxication. I guess he must like our hotel with its three square meals a day and soft warm bed at night."

I sense that something more bothering Fred. "How can I help you?"

He stands up and begins to pace. "My decision to evacuate the blood clot on his brain was easy. There wasn't any way for me to get consent, but since I felt the surgery was an emergency, I had no choice. I used my signature and asked the intensivist to countersign the consent form for surgery." He looks up and adds, "I'm grateful that California law supports urgent treatment in emergency situations."

He stops and stands in front of me. "I'd like your input to help guide the direction of his further care. I don't need to tell you that his prognosis is terrible. Here is my question: Do I have to continue active treatment no matter what complications develop?"

Fred stares at Mr. Phillips room. "When, if ever, could I justify switching him to comfort care? I don't want to make that call on my own."

I see a wry smile on his face as he continues with a thought I frequently ruminate over myself, "Looks like I have to add this to the information that they didn't teach me about during my medical training."

I sigh as I realize that little has changed since I graduated from medical school nearly fifty years ago. It seems that basic medical sciences and the ability to diagnose and treat endless diseases continue to take precedence over learning how to balance the benefits and burdens of these treatments. We only really begin to learn how to administer end of life care after we enter the arena of active medical practice. This is when we have the luxury of knowing our patients over a long period of time. Then, we realize that there is more to our patient than his chief complaint, diagnosis, or abnormal laboratory tests.

I spend the next quarter hour scanning Mr. Phillips' EMR. I count the number of admissions listed in his chart. During the four years that we have had computerized records, he racked up ten hospitalizations and sixty-two ER visits. All of these had been for complications of acute and chronic alcoholism: DT's, pneumonia, seizures, and malnutrition. He spends more time in our hospital than on the street.

I check his last two admissions more closely. I discover that several months ago one of the nurses noted that Mr. Phillip's told her, "All of my life I have been drinking more than two pints of vodka a day. I'm going to stop drinking. I need another drink like I need a shot in my head."

She also reported that his mind appeared clear when he told her that he would like a full attempt at resuscitation if he had a cardiac arrest. He said he didn't mind spending the rest of his life in a skilled nursing facility if it came down to that. However, he added that he did not want prolonged life support if it wouldn't help him leave the hospital.

Those reports make it apparent to me that Mr. Phillips recognized the depth of his illness. Ultimately, his long history of readmissions and visits for excessive alcoholism showed he didn't have the ability to control his addiction like he wished he could.

The most important information was his verbal statement that he wanted us to attempt cardiac resuscitation if his heart were to stop but he didn't want prolonged life support measures if they were unlikely to allow him to be discharged from the hospital. However, since his comments were not written as an Advance Health Care Directive[1], they were only legally binding for that specific admission. At the same time, they give Fred and me an important insight into his thoughts regarding his end of life care.

Mr. Phillips' current hospitalization record reports comments by both the neurosurgeon and the intensivist that his neurological findings are irreversible. The chance of any meaningful recovery is nil.

I turn off the computer and page Fred so I can discuss my findings with him and show him the documentation I found on the earlier record.

Dr. Fred Wright agrees that Mr. Phillips would most likely not want to continue active treatment in view of his prognosis. He changes his goal of therapy for him from curative measures to comfort care. He writes a "Do Not Attempt Resuscitation" order in the case of cardiac arrest. He then transfers Mr. Phillips from the intensive care unit to the general medical floor where the nursing staff gives him narcotics, anticholinergics, and sedatives for comfort. Mr. Phillips receives daily visits from a chaplain from the Spiritual Care Department as well as from a member of the hospital's *No One Dies Alone* program, a team of volunteers who sit with dying patients. Charlie Phillips never regains consciousness. He expires six days later.

Reflections
Capacity

The patient's ability to understand and respond to a specific question at a given time determines his mental capacity. In California, the courts do not decide on medical capacity. State law presumes that a patient has capacity[2] to make medical decisions unless a physician demonstrates otherwise.

One's level of capacity will depend on the questions that are asked. For example, a mentally challenged patient could have the capacity to appoint a surrogate decision-maker, but not to be able to decide on complex therapy.

There are ways to maximize the patient's facility to respond to the questions asked. Medical personnel could do well to take into account the time of day or night the patient is more awake. It is also wise to note the need to regulate external impediments such as noise or light and to adjust the timing of mind-numbing medications. Even slight improvement of mental status may allow the patient to express his own wishes about the extent of his medical care.

Both the physician and family can assess the following areas in determining a patient's capacity for informed consent[3] by noticing if the patient:

- *Understands what is wrong and what the proposed treatments are?*
- *Appreciates the benefits and risks of different proposed treatments or failure to treat?*
- *Discerns the medical information and relates this information to his personal values?*
- *Expresses his wishes and is able to communicate them?*

In circumstances where the doctor feels he lacks expertise in determining capacity, he can obtain a psychological consultation. In rare situations, the courts can step in to determine a patient's global competency or incompetency. However, because this process is both costly and lengthy, the legal profession prefers physicians to handle capacity issues in the hospital. In difficult cases, the physician or family may want to ask the hospital's bioethics committee for advice.

Mr. Phillips lacked the capacity to make medical decisions during his entire hospitalization. He did not have a surrogate to make those decisions for him. Therefore, the medical staff had the obligation to make decisions according to Mr. Phillips' best interests.

The medical record is a living document with copious documentation. Physicians often ignore previous hospitalization records because they are difficult to locate, and when found, are often voluminous. The plethora of routine data buried in the chart may contain unexpected important findings. I hope that future versions of the electronic medical record will speak to this problem and allow for easy retrieval of information to help streamline future care of our patients.

Mr. Phillips' case is one where we were able to utilize the *retrospectoscope* when we reviewed the records of his prior hospitalization. This apparatus is an ethereal medical instrument that we all use in medicine, but cannot find in our little black bags. We find it packaged with reflection upon our own experience and up to date knowledge. The *retro* portion allows us to look back on the patient's past experiences. This allows us to discover easily missed clues. When consulting on a patient, I have occasionally found statements in older records that clarified our patient's desires and enlightened the direction of treatment.

It is difficult for an extremely ill patient to think in complex detail when asked if he has any questions. His response may simply be:

- *Am I going to die?*
- *How long do I have left to live?*
- *Can you cure me?*
- *Can you take away my pain?*

When we hear these questions we have an opportunity to answer them with simplicity and truth. This can lead to more in depth discussions regarding the patient's wishes and stand a better chance of directing his care. I find even if a patient enters the hospital alert and oriented, he may develop confusion as his illness deteriorates. This is more reason to discuss the issues early upon admission.

Dr. Fred Wright did not have to make decisions without some knowledge of Mr. Phillips' wishes. The discovery of his patient's earlier comments clarified the course of treatment. He was finally at ease to direct his treatment to comfort care. Lacking that knowledge, Dr. Wright might have felt obligated to continue active and futile treatment, something that Mr. Phillips would not have wanted.

---

1. Chapter 9 *"Listen to Me!"* (Advance Health Care Directive)
2. Cal. Prob. Codes § 4657 and 4658
3. Chapter 17: *Further Reflections* (Informed Consent)

8
Who's on First?
Surrogacy

Tim Harper is forty-five. He has multiple medical problems including cortical blindness, seizures and a history of a head trauma that left him with severe injury to his brain. Presently, he suffers from diabetes, a large infected sacral ulceration, and chronic renal failure requiring dialysis. His two relatives live in other counties and both want to be Mr. Harper's surrogate decision-maker. However, they differ on his code status and goals of treatment.

It is Tuesday morning. Janie Britten, our social worker on the general medical floor, is on the phone with me. I am surprised to hear her voice this early in the week. I remind her that most of her ethical referrals occur late Friday afternoons, just before the staff leaves the hospital for the weekend.

"Hi, Janie, what can I do for you?"

"I've got a family situation over here and I can use your help."

She tells me the story in her usual clipped clinical fashion. "Tim Harper suffered a traumatic brain injury when he was eighteen. That was twenty-seven years ago. His foster mother has given him one-on-one care, twenty-four/seven, since his accident."

Janie pauses for a moment. "She died of cancer last week. Over the past few months, Mr. Harper's mental status has decreased from his already compromised baseline state. He came into the hospital a few days ago after having a prolonged seizure."

56

WE CAN, BUT SHOULD WE?

I detect some frustration in her voice as she approaches the core of the difficulty. "The only relatives I can locate are an aunt, Trudy, in Sacramento and his foster sister, Penny, in San Diego. I talked with each of them and both are willing to act as surrogate decision-makers. The problem is that they have different treatment goals in mind.

Janie relates her concerns. "His foster mother had neglected to appoint a surrogate for her son when she faced her own terminal illness. Now these decisions are left for these two family members who have had little contact with him over the years."

"I hope that these two women will work together for the patient's wellbeing once they are apprised of Mr. Harper's condition. What does your intuition tell you about them?"

"Well, neither of them has visited Mr. Harper for several years, but they seem serious about stepping up to the plate now that his foster mother has died. Trudy would like him to be placed in a nursing facility near Sacramento and be a No Code if his heart stops."

"What about Penny?"

"She would like to care for him in her home. She wants him to be a Full Code."

"Is the patient alert enough to give us any input on who he'd like to make these decisions?"

Janie sighs. "No. He's pretty confused. Both ladies tell me that he hasn't made any sense for a number of years."

I think for a moment and rephrase what I heard to be the primary ethical issue. "Okay, we have two people who want to be surrogates, but neither one has seen the patient for some time, and they don't agree about what should be done for Mr. Harper." I ask Janie, "Are they willing to speak to each other or do they seem entrenched in their own plans of care?"

"I doubt if they can come to an agreement between themselves. In fact, I don't know if they have spoken to each other about him."

"Sounds like we'll need a case conference with all the players. Can you set one up for tomorrow at 1:00?"

"Sure. I can ask Trudy to come here in person. Penny lives too far away. We'll need to patch her in by phone."

I am not happy with chairing a conference with a key person physically absent. It's difficult enough to facilitate these meetings between people who disagree when they're in the same room. Having one of them on the phone deprives everyone from making eye contact and from noting body language. "I hope they will be able to absorb the information in light of what is best for Mr. Harper."

We meet in the 4-North physical therapy storage room, the only space available for a meeting that afternoon. The hospitalist, palliative care physician, Janie, Trudy, Trudy's husband, and three foster siblings crowd into the small room. Penny, Penny's husband and another foster relative are on the phone. I begin the meeting after we introduce ourselves and make a sound-check of our voices to assure that we can hear each other over the telephone line.

The meeting lasts a bit over an hour and proves to be as difficult as I had feared. Penny has her own agenda and tends to dominate the conference. "Timmy is a good boy. I remember how much he liked playing with me when we were little. He loved hide and seek." She continues to talk in a rambling fashion, focusing on the past rather than the present. Trudy attempts to get a word in edgewise, but every time she begins a sentence, Penny interrupts.

As both of their voices begin to rise, I see we are not getting any closer to solving our dilemma. I speak above Penny's voice to redirect our attention. "Excuse me, Penny and Trudy, now it's time for us to hear from our physicians. They will explain Tim's current medical condition and his expected prognosis."

While the doctors lay out Mr. Harper's situation, I see Trudy's surprise and concern deepen. The hospitalist points out, "His mental status and kidney function are deteriorating. The large ulcer on his back is infected. He is unable to swallow food and requires a feeding tube for nutritional support."

The palliative care physician tells us about the benefits and burdens of code status options and dialysis. He reports, "Mr. Harper pulled out several nasal feeding tubes within a day of placement. Because he has a bleeding disorder that could cause a hemorrhage, we cannot place a feeding tube through his abdomen into his intestinal tract." He makes his prognosis clear, "Mr. Harper will never be capable of caring for himself, and, much less, ambulate on his own. He will require total care for the rest of his life."

58

WE CAN, BUT SHOULD WE?

I look at Trudy as I describe what total care means. "Someone will have to be with Tim every moment of the day and night. He will require help in going to the toilet, in bathing, feeding, caring for the large ulceration in his skin: his fragile skin must be protected from trauma. A physician or nurse must evaluate him on a regular basis which means making appointments and arranging for travel to and from the doctor's office."

Penny doesn't appear to understand the severity of her foster brother's medical condition. She insists, "I know I haven't seen Timmy for a number of years, but I'm certain he will get better with me. I live in an ideal setting. The weather is warm. My house is on a one-acre plot of grass with concrete walkways and flowers. I can wheel him out in a chair every day so he can see the sun and the birds. All he needs is love. I can care for him better than a skilled nursing home. I don't want my brother to die. There is a large medical center less than a mile from my home where he can go if he has an emergency."

Trudy speaks up. "Penny, you're wrong. I'm here. I can see how he looks. There's no way you or I have the ability to care for him. I want Timmy to go to a nursing home where he could get proper care. More important, if his heart stops, I want God to take him home."

Penny breaks in, "No, I want Timmy's heart to keep beating. Do everything to keep him alive."

It becomes obvious to me that if Penny were to have a role to play with Tim, she and her husband must visit him in the hospital to see his condition for themselves. When asked when she could come to the hospital, she responds, "We're too busy at this moment, but I can make decisions from down here." I repress the urge to wonder aloud how she would be able to care for him countless hours a week on an ongoing basis if she can't find the time to visit him in the hospital when he is critical.

By now, we have input from the doctors and family members. We are at an impasse between Trudy and Penny. I swallow and take a moment to think what to offer next. "I hear that both of you have Tim's best interests in mind. However, you both disagree regarding his long-term placement and care. So today we will focus on his present acute hospital care. Where he goes upon the doctor's discharge can be worked out later."

Trudy nods her head in agreement as Penny says, "I understand."

"We all agree that it is important for us to do what we think Tim would want if he could speak for himself. Presently, while he is in Northern California, Trudy can be the surrogate decision-maker since she lives only a bit more than an hour away. If and when he goes to San Diego, then Penny can be the surrogate. Can the two of you accept that as a compromise?"

I relax when they both answer, "Yes, doctor."

I breathe a sigh of relief and bring the meeting to a close.

Following the case conference, Trudy and the physicians change Tim's code status to Do Not Attempt Resuscitation if his heart were to stop. He has a slight improvement in his mental status over the next few days. However, he soon develops further decline in his functional status.

Mr. Harper remains in the hospital a total of five weeks. Throughout the hospitalization he varies between somnolence and agitation. The doctors eventually stop dialysis, as it does not help his renal failure. He pulls out his nasal feeding tube multiple times. After discussing the problem with Tim's physician, Trudy elects not to have a surgically placed tube inserted. She asks the physicians to change her nephew's goal of treatment to that of providing comfort. At that point, he no longer requires further acute hospital care.

Tim is transferred to a nursing home for end of life care with hospice support. He dies peacefully in less than a week.

Reflections
Surrogacy

Persons with mental capacity have the right to make their own medical decisions. When an adult patient lacks mental capacity on a permanent basis, the issue of surrogacy is most important in deciding appropriate care.

Mr. Harper's foster mother was his de facto surrogate even though she did not have legal standing from the courts. It would have been helpful when she discovered she had terminal cancer if she had arranged for a relative to have court appointed guardianship over her foster son or a written document expressing her wishes for his future care.

Ideally, we should all designate someone to be our healthcare agent by completing an Advance Health Care Document[1]. If we have not completed this form and are in the hospital, we can designate a surrogate by informing a member of the hospital staff who we would like to be our agent. However, when the doctor transcribes this information into our medical record, it will be valid *solely* for that hospitalization.

When necessary, it is best that the physician designate *one* person to be the patient's surrogate. Complications may arise when two or more people, such as Trudy and Penny in this chapter or Mr. Guerrero's nine daughters in Chapter 10, *No Man is an Island*, find themselves in the position of speaking for the patient. Each party may have diametrically opposed opinions about therapy. This can lead to argument and even schism between family members.

Generally, if we lose capacity and don't have a surrogate agent while we are hospitalized, it is up to the physician to determine the most appropriate person to guide the direction of our care. Many states mandate a definite hierarchy for the doctor to follow such as: the patient's spouse; followed by an adult child; parent; adult sibling; significant other; or a friend. California law does not codify such a sequence at the time of this writing. In California, the physician chooses the person who is concerned for our welfare and has knowledge about our previously expressed preferences regarding treatment. Appropriate surrogates[2] must:

- *Be in the best position to know our preferences.*
- *Be concerned for our welfare.*
- *Have expressed an interest in us by visits or inquiries during hospital stay.*

Even if a surrogate has been appointed, the physician can reject[3] a possible surrogate if:

- There are *reasons of conscience.*
- The surrogate makes *requests contrary to hospital policy.*
- The surrogate makes *requests for medically ineffective health care.*

J. Michael Gospe, M.D.

- The surrogate makes *requests for care contrary to medically acceptable health care standards.*

The surrogate's decisions must be in the patient's best interests[4] when considering:

- The patient's *relief of suffering.*
- The patient's *preservation of function.*
- The patient's *quality and extent of sustained life.*
- The *degree of intrusiveness, risk, or discomfort of treatment* to the patient.
- The *impact on those closest to the patient.*

In our current case, neither Trudy nor Penny fulfilled the above criteria for being an ideal surrogate. Mr. Harper's patient care conference[5] with physicians, staff, and family listened to all parties. This aided in arriving at a compromise. His present care was directed toward his current condition. His future care depended upon his progress.

Where there is opposition regarding available treatment, the chair of an ethical conference must remain neutral. The skill of active listening[6], coupled with respect toward all speakers, can help change a no-win situation into a win-win for the patient and surrogate. When the facilitator restates the position held by each participant, he shows he is paying attention to that person, all the while observing the speaker's facial expressions and body language. The facilitator may ask: *I notice you seem concerned. Do you have anything to add?* Questions like this promote dialogue rather than one individual *overriding* the goal of sharing information.

Difficulties arise when uncontrolled tension fills the room as they did at this meeting. A compromise developed only when both parties agreed to adjust their demands once all voices had been heard.

The facilitator and all participants must be reminded of their purpose: they are gathered together in order to listen with intent to create a plan that is best for the patient. Hopefully, this would be in a way the patient would want if he could speak for himself.

We must always remember that the patient comes first.

---

1. Chapter 9: *"Listen to Me!"* (Advance Health Care Document)
2. Barber v. Superior Court 1983

WE CAN, BUT SHOULD WE?

3. Cal. Prob. Code §4734-5
4. Barbers v Superior Court, 147 Cal. App. 3d 1006 (Cal. App. 1983)
5. Chapter 11: *"I Love My Son"* (Case Conferences)
6. Chapter 17: *Further Reflections* (Active Listening)

9
"Listen To Me!"
Advance Health Care Directive

Jack Barnard is sixty-six. His suffers from end-stage alcoholic liver disease complicated by portal hypertension, massive ascites, and hepatic encephalopathy. His Advance Health Care Directive (AHCD) states that he wishes to receive palliative care and comfort management. His wife, his appointed surrogate, demands further curative treatment of his liver disease.

Tyrone Brownstone is examining a patient in the intensive care unit and motions for me to come over. "I've got another one for you, Mike." Tyrone points to his patient, a man with massive ascites and canary yellow skin. "Lets go over to the nurses' break-room and steal a cup of coffee. I want to tell you about my problem."

The pot is constantly on simmer so there is only a slim chance that the coffee will be fresh. However, the nurses generally have an unlimited supply of cookies. After we pour our coffee and I locate a large chocolate chip cookie, I ask, "What's up, Ty?"

"This is really unusual for me. Even though he's unconscious, I know exactly what my patient wants and what he does not want us to do for him. Not only is there a copy of his Advance Health Care Directive in the chart, but also it is the most specific one I have ever seen. I know he wants us to get hospice involved, control his pain, and let him pass away in comfort."

WE CAN, BUT SHOULD WE?

I furrow my brow. "So, what's wrong with that?" The java was so thick and bitter I add cream and sugar into the brew, pick up a tongue blade to swirl the mixture, and wait for Ty to say more.

Ty takes a sip of coffee and reaches for a macaroon. "His wife is his designated surrogate. She wants to continue with full curative treatment, all stops out, go for broke."

"Ah. Therein lies the rub. Tell me more about your patient."

"Mr. Barnard is in his mid sixties. His body appears twenty or thirty years older because of the abuse he has given it. He was in Viet Nam in the sixties. He started drugs and alcohol when he was in the jungle and, although he eventually was able to get off the drug habit, he couldn't shake the booze."

This fits the man I see through the break-room doorway. His skin color is a brilliant yellow. His abdomen rises as though he is hiding a basketball under the covers. "Even looking at him from the hall, I can see he is nearing the end of the road."

"Yeah. He has rock hard cirrhosis, seizures, and a history of repeated esophageal bleeds from his portal hypertension. On top of that, he has COPD and smoked up to a week ago. The man arrived in the ER gasping with shallow and inefficient breathing. He was in a coma due to hepatic encephalopathy and didn't respond to deep pain when the ER doc poked him.

The ambulance crew brought in his directive. Someone had taped it to the fridge in his kitchen. In it he said he wanted to be a No Code and to have hospice called in if he were near death."

"What does his wife have to say?"

"That's the weird part. At first she asked that we do not intubate him under any circumstances and she agreed to have us connect her with hospice. Then, she demanded antibiotics, fluids, and a full court press. Her change of mind doesn't make any sense."

"Ty. Give me some time to review his chart and I'll get back to you. I wouldn't be surprised if we will need a case conference with his wife present. I find that when a surrogate goes against the patient's directive, a meeting with the doctor, nurse, and chaplain can often help clarify the surrogate's concerns."

J. Michael Gospe, M.D.

I peruse the documents. Mr. Bernard's Advance Health Care Directive is clear and concise. It is dated four months earlier. In it he states:

I would not want to have the following life sustaining treatments:

1. *If I am unconscious, in a coma or in a persistent vegetative state and there is little or no chance of recovery.*
2. *If I have permanent severe brain damage, for example severe dementia, which makes me unable to recognize my family or friends.*
3. *If I have a permanent condition that causes me to be completely dependent on others for my daily needs, for example eating, bathing, and toileting.*
4. *If I am confined to bed and need a breathing machine for the rest of my life.*
5. *If I have a condition that causes me to die very soon, even with life sustaining treatments.*
6. *If I have pain or other severe symptoms that cannot be relieved, it would depend on the circumstances.*

He then goes on to list the types of treatment he did not want including intubation, artificial nutrition, and attempted cardiac resuscitation.

I review his Veterans Administration Hospital records of a hospitalization only one month before. In that record, a physician wrote: *He states that he does not want to spend another day in the hospital and would rather die than take medications that will cause diarrhea.* That same note recorded that both the patient and his surrogate agreed to obtain hospice services at home.

After I complete my review of Mr. Barnard's records, I ask our social worker to set up a case conference in the 1-Center Conference Room for the next day.

Shortly after I dictate my note, the hospital's Palliative Care Nurse, Amanda Wand, meets with Mrs. Barnard. After their visit, Amanda tells me about their conversation.

"Mrs. Barnard is frightened about losing her husband. She cannot imagine being alone without him at her side. They married nearly twenty years ago and have no children. Mrs. Bernard watched her

66

husband's illness affect him over time. She said, 'My husband became sicker and sicker by the week. More than once, he told me his life was becoming too hard for him to tolerate. Now I cannot let him go.'"

Amanda continues, "After reading through Mr. Bernard's Advance Directive with her, I pointed out that he gave his physicians specific orders about what he wanted done for him should his present therapies stop working. His wishes are for a comfortable death." Amanda added, "I told her she didn't have to make that decision for him as he has already done it for himself and for her."

Hearing this, Mrs. Bernard agrees with her husband's physician to discharge her husband into hospice care at home. The conference is no longer necessary.

Reflections
Advance Health Care Directive

It is extremely difficult to decide life-changing issues for another person who has lost the ability to speak for himself. Under these circumstances, we need to honor what the patient would or would not want done for him, not what we would want for ourselves. This is where an Advance Health Care Document (AHCD) comes into the picture. It allows each of us to express our specific wishes concerning who[1] we want to speak for us if we no longer have the capacity to express our thoughts. It also allows us to specify our desires regarding our own end of life care. The document is legally binding and does not require a lawyer, although many attorneys include it when making wills for their clients. It is available at hospitals, many primary physicians' offices, law offices, and on the Internet.

An acute trauma, sudden stroke, massive heart attack, or even the expected deterioration of a chronic disease like Mr. Bernard's can alter our mental capacity in an instant. One moment we are active and alert, the next we are unconscious, sliding down a steep spiral into a coma. This places the burden of making decisions on our surrogate or family.

It is not unusual for patients with a chronic disease coupled with numerous stays in an intensive care unit to develop specifics regarding their own end of life care. After several courses of painful and unproductive therapy, many patients might elect to die peacefully rather than go through another round of invasive care. On the other hand, others may want extend their life even if that treatment is unlikely to succeed.

Most of the time, the patient will choose a surrogate to act when he or she no longer has the ability to communicate with the medical team. On rare occasions when a patient is overwhelmed with suffering or has a limited ability to speak or understand the English language, as with Mr. Guerrero in Chapter 10, *No Man is an Island*, he may choose that his surrogate receive information and decide for him while he still has the capacity to speak for himself.

In our present chapter, Mr. Bernard left a thoughtful and complete Advance Health Care Directive. His surrogate is legally bound to follow his wishes as written unless they are contrary to accepted medical practice or his current condition has changed significantly from what he was anticipating at the time he filled out the document. In those circumstances, the surrogate and attending physician have the obligation to modify Mr. Bernard's expressed wishes but to remain as true to them as possible.

You can see how an AHCD is an invaluable aide to the staff and family when dealing with discord. It clarifies the patient's goals because his wishes are known, clear and simple.

As the patient's condition worsens, the Advance Directive may remove the family's stress by supplying answers to common questions:

- *How long do we continue this treatment?*
- *What are the realistic options available?*
- *Is it certain this is the right time to terminate treatment?*
- *We cannot stop treatment; wouldn't that be killing him?*
- *What does comfort care involve?*

To answer these questions, the surrogate must understand the patient's present status in order to make a judgment regarding future medical care. Even with a legally filled-out document, it is often difficult for a surrogate to agree to the withdrawal of futile treatment when the patient expressed he did not want prolonged therapy.

When a surrogate agrees to comfort care or to withdraw treatment that results in death, s/he takes on a grave responsibility. It was only when Mrs. Bernard could see that her husband had made the decisions for himself that she could allow movement to honor his wishes. However, she could not do that until she could share her deepest doubts and fears with Amanda. Amanda listened. In turn, Amanda helped Mrs. Bernard hear her husband's desires; he wanted to die naturally, free from pain and suffering. Ultimately, she understood that her husband had already made his choice, that she was relieved of that responsibility.

An informative and supportive medical staff can go a long way toward achieving the common goal of honoring the patient's desires and easing the surrogate's stress. This underscores the wisdom of having persons on the team who are capable to respond to the concerns of the patient's loved ones.

I strongly believe it is up to the medical profession to encourage our chronically ill patients to complete an Advance Directive before they lose the capacity to speak for themselves. Primary care physicians and specialists including cardiologists, nephrologists, and oncologists are appropriate professionals to initiate a discussion about this document for vulnerable patients.

It would be ideal for all of us to complete a health care directive, to list *our* end of life wishes, and to select a person to act as *our* surrogate decision-maker should we become incapable of doing so. Acute trauma can affect anyone. Motor vehicle accidents, serious falls, and unexpected severe illness can occur any time in our life. The time to think about this issue is now. None of us are immune from death. We owe it to ourselves to be proactive in this matter. If you haven't already, I encourage you to begin your education now

---

1. Chapter 8: *Who's on First* (Surrogacy)

10
No Man is an Island
Communication

Jorge Guerrero is a seventy year-old farmworker with two possibly unrelated cancers: one in the lung, the other in the brain. Mr. and Mrs. Guerrero have been in this country for over thirty years. They do not speak English well. Consequently, adequate communication between the patient and members of the staff is flawed. Inadequate briefing between members of the staff has compounded the problem.

I stroll down the hospital corridor after attending a morning meeting. On this beautiful spring day, I daydream about being at our cabin and walking in the woods. Then, I notice Karen Minor, a Palliative Care nurse, staring at a computer screen in silence, her hands folded and brow furrowed.

"Is something wrong, Karen?"

She looks up and smiles. "I'm glad you're here, Mike. I visited a patient for a palliative consultation yesterday. His nurse asked me to see him again because of a devastating incident that occurred in his room less than an hour ago." She pauses for a moment.

I sit down next to her. "What happened?"

"Mr. Guerrero visited relatives in Mexico last week where he developed a urinary tract obstruction. A Mexican physician catheterized him and placed him on antibiotics. After he arrived home, he came to our emergency room for follow-up."

WE CAN, BUT SHOULD WE?

"Mr. Guerrero's daughter mentioned to the ER doc about her father's chronic cough and increased confusion over the past few months. A chest X-ray revealed a lung mass." Karen catches her breath, sighs, and continues. "He entered the hospital under a hospitalist, Dr. Harkens, who assumed his primary care."

"The next few days brought Mr. Guerrero one blow after another. A lung biopsy found that the mass was an aggressive Oat Cell Carcinoma. To top that off, the radiologists did an MRI of his head and discovered an abnormality in his brain. They're not sure if it's a metastasis from the lung or a primary brain tumor." She swallows, "It's so large the neurosurgeon says it is inoperable."

I think for a moment as I jot down a few notes. "That was a couple of days ago; what happened this morning?"

"First, I want to tell you about my visit yesterday." Karen stands, looks down the hallway, and turns toward me as she relives her visit. "Dr. Harkens asked me to see him. Rosa, the hospital's interpreter, and I arrived to find Mr. Guerrero's wife sitting next to his bed. She was crying and gripping his hand as if she would never let go. He lay in bed, silent, his eyes closed."

Karen goes on, "The two of them are overwhelmed with the torrent of medical information. They wanted further details to go through their children."

She shook her head. "I realized then how crucial the situation had become. With a sense of urgency, I posted their wishes in capital letters so that it would not be missed in his electronic medical chart."

Karen stops speaking for a second and I ask, "What happened then?"

"This morning, Dr. Jasper visited Mr. Guerrero for an Infectious Disease consultation. He went in without an interpreter and spoke to them in broken Spanish. He assumed they both knew the diagnoses. He told them Mr. Guerrero's fever came from an infection in his blood. He said that this, on top of the two cancers, made his prognosis dismal. He will probably die within weeks."

Karen takes a breath, "The Guerrero's son-in-law knew his wife's parents didn't want to hear all of this. He became unglued. He stood front of Dr. Jasper and yelled, 'Shut up.' Dr. Jasper shouted back. The head nurse had to call security to remove both men from the

71

room. That was when his nurse asked me to see if I could sooth the family's ruffled feathers.

"Fortunately, Rosa was available and we were able be at the bedside within minutes of the altercation. I wanted to cry when we entered. Mr. and Mrs. Guerrero were in shock. He was pale and breathing hard, wincing in pain with each gasp; his wife, sobbing, couldn't speak."

Karen's eyes blur with tears. I take in her distress and feel my stomach tighten. *This shouldn't have happened.* An interpreter would have facilitated Dr. Jasper's interactions with Mr. Guerrero and could have interceded before their conversation became explosive. Then, I ask myself, *Did Dr. Jasper read the last twenty-four hour postings of Mr. Guerrero's chart before seeing him? How well did he understand and speak Spanish?* Karen then told me "Dr. Jasper realized he made a mistake and removed himself from the case. He handed the infectious disease consultation over to his partner."

Karen brings me back to the present moment. "Mike, Mr. Guerrero is dying. He's confused. He's feeling pressured to do things he doesn't understand. He and his wife don't need this kind of stress on top of everything else they're facing."

I take a moment to ponder the situation. "Mr. Guerrero's current desires regarding any future health care decisions must be clarified to the entire team. Those in charge must be certain that they follow them twenty-four/seven. I'll arrange for a meeting between the Guerrero's, Dr. Harkens, and the staff for this afternoon. How does two o'clock work out for you?"

"That will be great. Thanks, Mike."

Mr. Guerrero's room is crowded as his family and caregivers surround his bed. While Rosa interprets for us, she positions herself out of sight to allow us to look directly at the speaker with her voice in the background. It reminds me of reading captions in a foreign movie. Before long, I feel all of us are speaking the same language.

After we introduce ourselves, I apologize to Mr. and Mrs. Guerrero for the events of the previous day. "We are here to communicate your wishes, Mr. Guerrero. Is it true that you do not want to be told anything more about your condition, its diagnosis, treatment possibilities, and eventual outcome?"

He looks directly into my eyes as he answers with a clear, "Si."

"Mrs. Guerrero, is this what you want as well?"

Her voice, barely a whisper, responds, "Si."

I turn my head back to the dying man in the bed. "Who would you like us to talk with? Who do you want to make your medical decisions?"

His answer is strong. "My daughters, all nine of them, together."

I pause for a moment. "Mr. Guerrero, we find it best that one of your daughters be named to speak with the doctors, then she can relay any information to the others as well as the family's decisions back to the doctors. Which of your daughters would be the best person to do this?"

I relax inside when he responds, "Make it my eldest daughter, Serena." Mrs. Guerrero sits quietly next to her husband; the fingers of her right hand intertwine with his; those of her left hand caress a well-worn rosary. She nods her head in agreement.

I turn my attention towards his children. With the exception of Serena's black hair that shows only a trace of gray, she is a clone of her mother. Both are short with round faces and deep brown eyes. At her father's words, she looks at him and appears to hold her breath.

"Serena, is this ok with you?"

"Yes, Doctor." Her voice is soft, but the words strong. Her English sports a veneer of an accent retained from her childhood in Puebla, Mexico.

"Mr. Guerrero, we would like to go to another room to discuss your treatment options. Any final decisions will be between Dr. Harkens and Serena. Is this what you want?"

"Si, Doctor." He is so exhausted he can barely keep his eyes open.

We all go to the conference room. I watch Serena's face as she listens to Doctor Harkens tell her about the benefits and burdens of obtaining a biopsy of the mass in her father's brain to determine whether it is a primary brain tumor or a metastasis. Her jaw tightens and her upper teeth pull her lower lip into her mouth. She says, "I think I understand what you are saying: my father's treatment will be different depending on what is causing the mass. Is that right?"

Dr. Harkens agrees and goes on to tell her about several forms of therapy that they can give Mr. Guerrero. "We can give active treatment with radiation and chemotherapy or switch the goal of treatment to comfort care. In that case, we would focus our efforts on making his last days more peaceful. There may even be the possibility of allowing him to visit Mexico one last time before he's incapable of making the trip. Under the best of circumstances, your father will only have six months to a year to live."

As the daughters hear what the he tells them, they sob and reach for the box of Kleenex near them. After the meeting, Dr. Harkens and I accompany Serena and her sisters back to their father's room. We tell Mr. Guerrero that he can return home after we perform several more tests.

Serena meets with her father's physician the next day. Further communication between Serena and the staff goes well. Mr. and Mrs. Guerrero rest in knowing their wishes are being acted upon.

Serena approves the doctors performing a brain biopsy on her father. Unfortunately, the procedure does not help clarify the situation as the slides reveal only dead cells. Because the MRI strongly suggests that the mass is a cancer, he undergoes a course of radiotherapy in an unsuccessful attempt to shrink the mass in his brain.

Mr. Guerrero lives at home with hospice support for three and one-half months before he passes away. He is confused most of that time, but fortunately, medication eases his pain and breathing difficulties.

Reflections
Communication

In my experience, inadequate communication is the root cause of the majority of ethical dilemmas in a hospital. The children's party game *telephone* points out how easy it is to garble and to misunderstand a simple oral message. Clear transmission of information is vital between all involved in a patient's medical care: the patient, family, and members of the hospital staff, including spiritual care. Complex details can be lost if not relayed simply, in ways that can be understood, in ways that invite questions.

As human beings, our culture, beliefs, traditions, and unique backgrounds meld together to form our personal values. We set goals based on our perceived experiences. As healthcare providers, we bring our unique history and medical knowledge together to work towards the best outcome for our patients.

Sometimes we forget that what seems to be a sensible approach from our medical standpoint may not be fitting or respectful of our patient's desires. This is especially true in a hospital setting where a patient's care lays in the hands of a variety of medical specialists. They each may forge ahead with a planned scenario and ignore their patient's and his family's inability to grasp more information, as it was true for Mr. Guerrero. Multiple new findings clouded his ability to receive detailed information in order to make informed decisions. The good news came after the shock Mr. and Mrs. Guerrero experienced at the time of their altercation with the infectious disease specialist. They were finally able to express their wishes regarding further knowledge about his disease. These wishes were honored in their entirety by the medical staff.

Medical professionals and family members can become more aware of their patient's or loved one's emotional state by gently approaching the bedside and making eye contact, rather than standing at the end of the bed and peering only at monitor screens. A touch goes a long way to ease a stressful moment.

As with the bold approach of Mr. Guerrero's infectious disease consultant, we may cause unnecessary stress that could have been avoided from our mistaken assumptions:

- *I assume my ability to speak Spanish does not warrant an interpreter.*
- *I assume he knows his latest diagnoses.*
- *I assume he wants to know everything about his disease.*
- *I assume he wants to make his own decisions.*
- *I assume he can take in what I am going to tell him.*

J. Michael Gospe, M.D.

The consultant's lack of awareness of Mr. Guerrero's emotional state caught the patient, his family, and staff at a pivotal moment. Once the palliative care nurse identified the problem, she sought mediation by the medical ethics team. The team interceded immediately by providing a space for Mr. Guerrero to voice his wishes in front of witnesses. The facilitated conference with professionals and family devised an appropriate care plan based on his desires.

When I think about Mr. and Mrs. Guerrero, I remember the poem "No Man is an Island" by John Donne:
No man is an island, entire of itself:
Every man is a piece of the continent, a part of the main.
Healthcare providers, patients, and families, please take Donne's poem to heart. Remember everyone involved with a patient's treatment has important information to share.

Clear, concise communication is crucial whether it is verbal, handwritten, or electronic. One-on-one interaction regarding changes in the patient's condition or his desires is imperative to increase efficiency, accuracy, and a better outcome. Most important, it can decrease a patient's anxiety. Without it, unnecessary burdens can build up and overpower the benefits of treatment. When the material is important enough, it bears *repeating* vocally.

Realistically, the majority of information shared by the hospital staff is not verbal. It is contained in the patient's medical record. Prolonged hospital stays with a variety of specialists noting observations and hourly nurses' notes produce an extremely dense medical record. This material is not a dialogue; it does not allow for the give and take of information. Unfortunately, it also may not point to older information that is still pertinent yet now lays buried.

Mr. Guerrero entered our hospital shortly after we began the use of an electronic medical record (EMR). Prior to that time, the handwritten bedside chart held this information. Colored sticky notes flagged crucial details, important questions, and answered inquiries for the staff to review as they began each shift. They were easy to see and simple to use. Now they are gone.

WE CAN, BUT SHOULD WE?

Other disadvantages come with the use of the EMR. Physicians tend to insert long and repetitive reports into the record. Mr. Guerrero's infectious disease doctor failed to see Karen's comments regarding the patient's wish for protection from further information concerning his diagnosis. It lay beneath other reports generated during this hospitalization. How many doctors take the time to read further back than the past twenty-four hour entries?

Presently, when a healthcare worker posts pertinent findings into the chart, s/he cannot assume the team members will read it. Thus eye-to-eye or mouth-to-ear transmission is crucial. When one-on-one communication fails or is not practical, I recommend consideration of a multidisciplinary case conference[1] early in a complex patient's hospital stay.

Our EMR does have some advantages over the paper chart and its handwritten notes. Decoding a doctor's handwriting sometimes propagates significant errors in translation. The newer computer-generated fonts improve the staff's ability to read each notation. In addition, the electronic format allows the reader to easily evaluate and analyze laboratory tests and X-ray findings.

I leave you with two quotations that sum up the difficulties we can experience when people do not listen with an open mind and an open heart.

Much unhappiness has come into the world
because of bewilderment and things left unsaid.
Fyodor Dostoyevsky

The single biggest problem in communication is
the illusion that it has taken place.
George Bernard Shaw

---

1. Chapter 11: *"I Love My Son"* (Case Conferences)

11
"I Love My Son"
Case Conferences

Fred Franklin is forty years old. He has been in an irreversible coma for three weeks following a bicycle-automobile accident. Both his wife and his physician want to terminate his active treatment and begin comfort care to allow him to die a natural death. Several members of Fred's family have conflicting views.

This November in Santa Rosa is extremely wet. Water fills the beds of nearby rivers and creeks and turns intersections into lakes and backyards into oceans. I am about to put on my raincoat and leave my office for home when my secretary calls.

"Mike, don't leave yet. Chris Johnson is on the phone for you."

I drape my slicker over the back of a chair and pick up the phone. "Hi, Chris. Wet enough for you?"

"You bet, Mike. Boy this weather is biblical. I've looked for the Ark, but haven't spotted it yet."

"I'm guessing you didn't call about the weather. What's up?"

"I've had one of my primary care patients in the hospital for three weeks. An ethical problem has been brewing for a while and it's coming to a head. I was hoping you could give me a hand."

"Give me a run-down. Is it urgent enough to see tonight, or would tomorrow work?"

"Tomorrow would be fine. I'd like to get this ironed out before the weekend." Chris continues. "Fred Franklin is an engineer at HP. He has the nicest wife and two young kids. They've been in my practice

78

for over ten years. Three weeks ago, Fred was biking on Petaluma Hill Road on his way home from work. The first storm hit just before he approached the spot where it makes a sharp upward turn."

"I stay away from that road. Even in good weather it scares me."

"Anyway, Fred was caught in the downpour when he was only a mile from home. His bike skidded and he crossed the line. A car coming down the road hit him. He's got a terrible brain injury. Looks like he's going to die any day now. His wife, who is a nurse, his neurosurgeon, and I all agree we should switch to comfort care. Fred's mother and sister insist on a full court press."

I sigh. "I'll drop by in the morning, take a look at him, and give you a buzz when I'm through."

"Thanks, Mike. Stay dry."

"You too, Chris."

Morning brings clear skies and the long awaited sun. It warms the soaked ground as well as my spirits. As I approach the ICU, I think about many of my patients who suffered severe brain injuries. I realize how difficult it is for their family to accept a dismal prognosis when their loved one appears to be in a deep comfortable sleep, as if he is waiting for the buzz of an alarm clock to wake him up.

I notice Sara Bailey, Fred Franklin's primary nurse, charting at the desk across from his room. Sara has been a regular in the ICU for almost as long as I have been on staff. She is a small vigorous lady in her fifties, smart and astute.

"Hi, Sara."

"Oh, hello, Mike. What can I do for you?"

"Chris Johnson asked me to look in on Mr. Franklin to consult on the rising ethical concern involving Mrs. Franklin and her in-laws. What's your take on the situation?"

Sara points to her patient's room. An elderly lady sits beside the bed. Sara motions me toward the nurses' break room. "Let's go in here where we can talk privately."

I follow her into a room nearby. We ignore a table that is decorated with a smattering of dirty dishes, used cups, a tray of donuts, and scattered paper napkins. We locate two chairs in a corner and Sara begins to tell me about Mr. Franklin.

J. Michael Gospe, M.D.

"I've cared for Fred much of the time he has been in the unit. I feel so sorry for his wife. Joan and I speak on the phone nearly every day. With her nursing background, she is able to understand Fred's injuries and his poor prognosis. Stress at home occupies a lot of her time, so she is unable to be here as much as she'd like. Their sixteen-year-old son, Jim, is recuperating from a motorcycle accident that occurred shortly before Fred's injury. Both Jim and his little sister, Amy, are having difficulty dealing with their father's serious condition. Joan is torn between her children's need for her presence and her need to be with her husband."

Sara looks through the doorway toward Fred's room across the hall. "On the other hand, Fred's mother, Ethel, poses a problem." Sara sighs. "Ethel came to town from Colorado with her daughter, Elizabeth, immediately after the accident. She hardly ever leaves Fred's room. She is angry with her daughter-in-law because Joan isn't in the hospital all day. Ethel wants to take Fred back to Colorado with her. She's convinced he'll recover faster in her home where he can enjoy her flower garden. I don't know where she gets that idea. Flower gardens can't grow in Colorado in the middle of winter. God, Ethel is in her own little world."

I stand up, take a deep breath, and turn toward the patient's room. "Time for me to bite the bullet, see Fred, and meet his mother."

"Good luck, Doc. You'll need it."

It is too easy to look at Ethel as an obstructive person who is refusing to follow Fred's doctors' advice. I tell my self to remember that she is suffering as much as Joan. Ethel cannot bear to see her son taken away from her.

"Hello, Mrs. Franklin. I'm Dr. Gospe. I'm the Chair of the hospital's ethics committee. Dr. Johnson asked me to visit Fred. He has requested a meeting between your family and the doctors so we can discuss the various options available for Fred's further care."

Tears fill Ethel's eyes. She puts down her knitting and looks up at me. I feel her grief as she says, "I know my son will wake up any moment. I want to look after Fred at my house until he recovers. He cannot die. His father passed fifteen years ago and I am so lonely." She sobs and buries her face in a worn handkerchief. "Joan, the

80

doctors, and nurses are all pushing to have Fred's life support removed. I don't want them to kill my son. Doctor, please help me save him."

Ethel's pronouncements touch me. She would move heaven and earth to make everything better. I also understand the position that Joan and the doctors are taking in view of Fred's prognosis. This is a true dilemma with two directly opposite directions that Mr. Franklin's treatment might take. It is important for me to keep an open mind and listen to everyone.

I take a seat next to Ethel and speak softly to her. "Mrs. Franklin, our aim is to do everything within our power to help Fred. I'm going to set up a meeting between all of us for tomorrow at 3:00. I will ask Ms. Scott, our social worker, to make the arrangements and contact everyone. She will check with you and Joan to see if other family members wish to be invited."

As I leave Fred's room, I look at the gauges on the machines attached to him. Oxygen and a number of drugs keep his body stable in his comatose state. The neurosurgical notes in his chart report he is functioning at a basic level; his brain will not recover from the injuries he received from the accident.

The small conference room is crowded with ten of us. There are three physicians: Fred's neurosurgeon Betty O'Keefe, Chris, and me. Sara and Helen round out the staff at the meeting. Joan, her son, Jim, and their minister, Howard Dunn, sit next to a window. Fred's sister, Elizabeth Reyes, and Ethel take seats by the door. I notice Ethel take her knitting out of her purse. She avoids making eye contact with Joan.

I ask the participants to introduce themselves and then set the ground rules. "The purpose of this meeting is to allow us to discuss the options available for Fred. He does not have an Advance Healthcare Directive and has not appointed a surrogate decision-maker. However, Joan and Fred have been married for over twenty years. She is the appropriate person to speak for Fred since he cannot speak for himself. All of us will have an opportunity to speak. Any final decisions concerning Fred's care will be between Joan and Dr. Johnson."

Joan sighs and nods her head. Ethel clenches her jaw while Elizabeth squirms in her seat. Jim appears oblivious to what is going on in the room as he focuses on the game he is playing on his Game Boy computer.

I ask Joan to give us her understanding of Fred's current condition and prognosis.

Joan reaches for a tissue as she speaks. "I know Fred is dying. His damaged brain is beyond repair; he's in a permanent coma. The doctors are consistent in the information they give me and, as a nurse, I realize the machines burden his body far more than any benefits they give him." Her voice breaks. "I don't want my husband to die but I don't want him to suffer needlessly."

She continues, "My children are confused and don't understand their father's condition. Jim shattered his leg six weeks ago from a motorcycle accident. After three weeks in the hospital, he is now recovering at home. Amy's fifth grade school work is suffering. She can't sleep. She is worried and bewildered."

Joan pauses for a moment to collect her thoughts. "Elizabeth and Ethel don't think Fred's as bad as the doctors are telling us. They want us to continue treating him the way we are. I know we'll eventually lose Fred and I'm torn between letting him go or possibly destroying the relationship between the rest of the family and me."

I thank Joan and pause for a moment. Then, I turn toward Dr. O'Keefe, "Betty, will you please bring us up to date with Fred's neurological status."

Betty speaks clearly, with compassion in her New York accent. "Fred has a condition we call a Persistent Vegetative State. He has basic reflexes but his thinking processes have died. His eyes are open, but his brain doesn't work. He may look like he is awake, but I'm afraid all he can do is breathe and blink. He cannot respond to external stimuli. He will never be Fred again." She looks directly at Joan and then turns toward Ethel and Elizabeth. "If Fred is able to survive, he will not be able to care for himself."

Chris speaks up. "On top of Fred's coma, many of his body systems are failing. He has pneumonia, an infection in his blood stream, very low blood pressure, and kidney damage. I agree with Dr.

WE CAN, BUT SHOULD WE?

O'Keefe that further active therapy will not reverse Fred's deteriorating condition. He will die soon no matter what we do."

I nod at our social worker. "Helen, what can you tell us about Fred's needs after hospitalization."

She responds, "Should Fred be well enough to leave the hospital, he will require around the clock skilled nursing care. Frequent changes in his position are necessary to keep his skin from developing ulcerations that could promote a severe infection. It is unlikely that the family could provide that at home. He would be best served in a long term nursing hospital."

I see Ethel shake her head in disbelief. She breathes rapidly and seems angry. "Mrs. Franklin, would you like to say something?"

Ethel looks around the room. "I am irate. You people don't know my son. I have been in the hospital ever since I got word about the accident. I see my son struggling every second of the day. He is a fighter. I know he understands everything that is happening to him. He wants to live." She peers at her daughter-in-law. "Joan, don't kill my son!"

Elizabeth stands up with anger flowing through her clenched teeth. "Fred is my big brother. He seems peaceful in bed. I can see him move his eyes and look at me when I come into the room. I grew up with him and he's not a quitter." She turns toward her sister-in-law. "Joan, I insist you let him live." Ethel nods approvingly while Joan quietly sobs.

I look over at Fred's son, Jim, sitting in a wheel chair next to his mother. He is a string bean adolescent wearing a heavy Erector Set contraption over his right leg, a result of the shattered bones followed by three extensive operations. He appears withdrawn but I see anger as he bites his upper lip.

"Jim," I ask, "You have been through a lot. Do you want to say anything?"

He mumbles. "Nope."

"Are you certain?"

"Yeah." Jim looks up from his computer game. "All I want to do is to get back to my team and play basketball." He slumps deeper in his chair. "Pull the plug; he's dead anyway."

"The last few weeks have been difficult for everyone. Pastor Dunn, I understand you have been spending time with Joan, Jim, and Amy throughout all of this. What are your thoughts?"

"I've known the family for a number of years. Fred and Joan are active in the choir and Fred is on the Church Council. I have been counseling them about their experiences as they go through this difficult time. They all seem to realize in their own way that death is not the end for Fred.

"I'm very concerned about the extraordinary stress that Joan has been under. She had to take a leave of absence from work. She feels torn between spending time with her children and her need to stay with Fred. Although the children don't understand the full extent of Fred's injuries, they realize that something very serious is about to happen to their father and their family."

Joan then breathes deeply and adds a new piece of information as if she just remembered it. "Last year I wrote a paper on end of life issues for my nursing Master's class. Fred did the typing for me and we had numerous discussions concerning our own desires for end of life care. He told me more than once that he never would want to live the way he is now. He would not want to be a burden. He would want to die in peace and with dignity."

A moment of stillness seems to honor this grief stricken family. Ethel stops knitting as she processes what she has just heard. She sighs; her body relaxes as if relieved. She turns toward her daughter-in-law. "Joan, I didn't know that." Her eyes begin to tear as she whispers, "If that's what my son wanted, then we must follow his wishes." Elizabeth quietly shakes her head in agreement.

Dr. Chris Johnson orders comfort care. Fred Franklin expires peacefully several days later.

Reflections
Case Conferences

Serious ethical situations can often be relieved by the utilization of a multidisciplinary case conference. These conferences are ways to develop better communication between patients, families, and staff by listening to concerns, reviewing the current status of the patient, and offering treatment options. In the present chapter we see how the presentation of new information allowed Fred Franklin's mother and sister to accept a change in his goal of therapy to comfort care. This knowledge reframed Fred's treatment plan. His truth punctured the wall of dissonance in the room. In Chapter 8, *Whose on* First, the staff and family are able to chose an appropriate surrogate for Tim Harper; in Chapter 10, *No Man is an Island*, Mr. and Mrs. Guerrero communicate their wishes to the appropriate staff members, and in Chapter 12, *Waiting...*, the Chen family and physician come to a compromise.

It is human nature to experience stress when faced with a life-changing diagnosis. In my gastroenterology practice, I made it a point never to give a serious diagnosis over the phone. I also suggested that my patient invite a family member to act as another pair of ears and eyes. I learned early on in my medical career that once the "C" word was mentioned, my patients rarely were able to take in any further information.

Since grief and stress commonly enshroud extremely ill hospitalized patients and their families, it is important for the medical team to empathize with them, to develop a compassionate attitude, to offer comfort, and to take time to explain what is happening in ways that the patient and loved ones can understand.

Even when this occurs, the medical team may become irritated when family members hold beliefs that lead to intractable goals for their loved one. Their annoyance can subtly grow into a serious medical dilemma if allowed to fester. Nipping this in the bud is the key here. A multidisciplinary case conference can offer a wider and non-judgmental landscape where time, patience, kindness, and listening on the part of the medical team can open a space where important facts and misconceptions may be absorbed. It can clear the air of discontent and denial and often results in all participants to better understand each other. This in time leads to improved care for the patient, who is the most important person here.

As we saw in Chapter 15, *Inevitable Death,* there are times when a case conference does not go the way we had hoped. I learned long ago not to have any preconceived expectations for a conference.

J. Michael Gospe, M.D.

Certainly, I do have specific areas I want covered such as Code Status or choices of a surrogate. However, each conference takes on its own life. We need to be flexible in order to come to a conclusion that is best for our specific patient.

Ethical case conferences may not be necessary if the staff is able to identify and explore potential ethical issues at an early onset. Clear communication[1] with active listening[2] on the part of the physicians, nurses, and families can identify early signs of and respond to the patient's non-verbal cues.

In Fred's situation, we see how Ethel and Elizabeth's lack of medical knowledge, coupled with fear of losing their son and brother, blinded them to the truth about his prognosis. They were given the opportunity to express their worries. When Fred spoke for himself through Joan, his mother and sister found a way to let Fred pass away in comfort.

After I consult on a case, I determine if a conference is necessary by reviewing the chart, visiting the patient and speaking to the appropriate members of the staff and family. If the problem cannot be resolved easily, I speak with the involved physicians and have them choose a date and time that fits their schedule. The social worker and I determine which staff members should attend. The social worker then invites the patient's support group and the patient, if he is capable to join us. An ideal number for a conference is between ten and twelve. More people make it difficult for everyone to have a chance to absorb the information and speak. Having fewer people does not allow a variety of information to be exchanged.

These meetings require nearly an hour. Conferences may be hard to arrange because of busy schedules. Sometimes it is difficult to convince physicians and staff members that such an hour is worthwhile. I stress the benefits of these meetings including a unification of goals, peace of mind, improved morale, and a more comfortable hospitalization for the patient. However, until insurance plans compensate the physician's time for these important meetings, I fear that the difficulties in having them attend case conferences will continue to be a stumbling block.

WE CAN, BUT SHOULD WE?

As facilitator for the group conference, I have a number of responsibilities that can improve the outcome of the meeting:

- *Review* the clinical facts.
- *Identify issues* of concern.
- *Emphasize* that any final treatment decisions will be between the physician and the patient or patient's surrogate decision-maker.
- *Allow* a discussion of all goals of treatment, available options, and possible solutions.
- *Be aware* of body language and identify personal feelings of the participants.
- *Give* the family time to process this information.
- *Arrange* for another meeting if necessary.

I attempt to improve any potential imbalance between the patient/family and staff. Because of the doctor's training, he or she is often thought of as having all of the answer. This can block the patient/family from expressing their thoughts. Because of this, I first ask the patient's loved ones to describe their understanding of the patient's condition, prognosis, and goals of therapy. This subtly flips the status pyramid on its head, giving needed weight to the patient and family's viewpoints. Next, I invite the medical staff to present their findings and establish a dialogue between participants. A sensitive, nonjudgmental, ethically oriented meeting of the patient's *community of concern* often clarifies issues that were previously unknown or felt to be insurmountable.

The medical team needs to be aware of their patient and family's worries as expressed both orally and through body language. They may not be able to find words to convey their concerns. They may not understand medical vocabulary. They may feel ignored when they ask for information regarding care or drugs. They may feel afraid to express questions such as what is the cause of his symptoms or comments on his goals of therapy. Their uneasiness could result in distrust of the professionals caring for him. Depression and hostility may follow. Once again, active listening invites chaos to move into order.

J. Michael Gospe, M.D.

Stories are a great teaching moment. For the past few years, I have used a synopsis of Fred's case as a basis for role-playing by nursing students at the local junior college. Debriefing after these sessions has been educational both to the students as well as to myself. We have all learned the importance of stepping into another's shoes and the importance of broadening our outlook and not assuming that *we* have all of the answers to difficult problems.

---

1. Chapter 10: *No Man is an Island* (Communication)
2. Chapter 17: *Further Reflections* (Active Listening)

12
Waiting ...
Cultural Conflicts

Hui Chen, is a seventy-eight year-old Filipino of Chinese ancestry with metastatic lung carcinoma and multi-system failure. He is unresponsive to stimuli and his physician wants to shift the goal of treatment to comfort care. The family refuses to make any change in the direction of his care until Mr. Chen's son returns from a Caribbean cruise.

It is eleven-thirty Friday morning. Doctor Ned Briggs sits quietly in front of one of the Intensive Care Unit computer terminals. Ned is a thoughtful and caring man with over twenty-five years of experience as an intensive care specialist. He wears a long white lab coat. A black stethoscope around his neck frames his closely cropped beard. His eyes scan data on the screen as his hands rest on the keyboard.

Ned looks up and mumbles, "I have been in this business a heck of a long time, but this one's really gotten to me. It's not fair. I can't continue to treat my patient this way."

"What's the matter, Ned?"

"I can really use your help, Mike." He swivels his chair to face me and invites me to sit next to him. He takes a breath. "I've got this man, Mr. Chen, who's circling the drain with a widespread cancer. His organs are shutting down. All the nurses, palliative team, chaplains, everyone agrees with me: we need to stop torturing him." Ned quietly strokes his beard and calms down. "I don't know if he's feeling pain, but those blood sticks have got to be uncomfortable. The lab results show the drugs we're pumping into him aren't making him any better. His numbers are bottoming out: blood pressure, hemoglobin, kidney function; they all stink."

"If it's so clear, why not switch your goal of treatment to comfort care?"

"The family won't let me." Ned clenches his jaw. "His eldest daughter insists we wait until their brother arrives. He is the patient's only son. She says he is the only one who can make the decision to withdraw care. I've lost count of how many times I went over everything with her, but she won't change her mind."

I understand his discomfort. It is always frustrating when a family insists on ineffectual treatment and refuses to follow their doctor's recommendation to discontinue it. Add a physician's moral compunction of burdening his patient needlessly, and we have a crucial situation. "Where is the son? Can you get him on the phone?"

Ned shakes his head. "God only knows; I sure don't. The daughter claims her brother is on a cruise ship somewhere in the Caribbean and either can't or won't get him to contact us. She keeps promising he'll return Monday." He lowers his voice. "That will be another four days of hell for my patient. I've had it with this family."

I put Ned's information into perspective. There is always more than one viewpoint to every medical dilemma. Although Ned's concerns are serious, I know it is necessary for us to look at all sides of the issue before we can reach the best answer for Mr. Chen.

"Ned, What do you think about having a case conference with the family? If we can get everyone together, we might be able to arrive at a compromise."

"Could be worth a try."

I look around the ICU and see Betty Limpet, an ICU social worker. "Betty will arrange for a meeting between the staff and family." Ned appears more relaxed as I ask him, "Are you free for a meeting this afternoon?" I look at my watch, "It's nine, how does three o'clock sound?"

"Yeah. That's ok. I'm stuck here all day anyway."

"I'll set it up in the ICU Conference Room."

WE CAN, BUT SHOULD WE?

I arrive at the conference room shortly before three. I estimate that eleven or twelve people will attend. The small room contains four couches able to hold up to ten people. To be sure there is enough seating, I bring in another three chairs from the hall and place them along the room's periphery in an inclusive circular fashion.

Shortly after three, the staff arrive: Doctor Briggs, Betty Limpet, Mr. Chen's nurse, a palliative care nurse, a student nurse, and the chaplain. The minutes tick by without the Chen family's arrival. I am about to call the meeting off when an elderly Asian woman enters the room with three younger women. I notice they set themselves apart from the staff as they squeeze together on an empty couch.

We introduce ourselves. Lily Wong, Mr. Chen's eldest daughter, speaks. She is a dignified lady with gray hair pulled back in a bun. In strong and firm Chinese accent, she informs us, "My mother does not understand English. She does not want to attend this meeting. I will speak for my mother and my two sisters." Her voice fills the room. "Don't you dare let our father die!" She pauses. "You must wait until our brother, Samuel, returns from his cruise." Her two sisters nod their heads in agreement as she continues, "I've told you all week that in our culture all major medical decisions must be made by a sick parent's oldest son. Samuel is our only brother. Our father would want him to be here and so do we." She pauses and looks at her family as her voice softens. "I know I'm speaking for everyone at this time. I cannot and will not make these decisions. My brother must do that."

I ask her, "Does your brother know about your father's condition and how serious it is?"

"Yes, Doctor. I emailed one of our relatives in Minnesota and she got through to Samuel on Facebook. He told her he would be here late Sunday night."

"Please contact your relative immediately. Ask her to send an urgent message to your brother. He must speak to Dr. Briggs as soon as possible. We should be able to get through to him with ship-to-shore radio or possibly Skype." I pause for a moment. "Otherwise, he could contact the hospital at the next port of call. Then he could discuss the case with your father's physician."

J. Michael Gospe, M.D.

Mrs. Wong's voice is steady as she repeats what she had previously told the doctor and social worker, "I don't know what cruise line he is on, the name of his ship, or his itinerary. All I know is that he is in the Caribbean and will be home as soon as he can. No, there is absolutely no way for the doctors to contact him." I see Ned becoming more agitated as she continues, "I don't want any changes made until Samuel arrives."

Hostility fills the room between the family and staff. It is as if Mrs. Wong has not heard any of the information the doctors shared with her over the course of her father's illness. And it is clear the staff has not heard the depths of her concerns.

I hope the family will be capable of understanding the seriousness of Mr. Chen's prognosis during this meeting. I turn to Ned. "Dr. Briggs, please tell us about Mr. Chen's current status."

Ned holds his anger in check as he brings the family up to date. "Your father has had lung cancer for five years. At first he responded to radiation and chemotherapy, but in this last year these treatments stopped working and the tumor is growing. Over the past week, I have watched him steadily deteriorate. He is now in a coma, his blood pressure is very low, and his kidneys and liver are shutting down." Ned's hands clench as he looks at Mrs. Wong. "Even worse, his brain function is nearly gone. Yesterday, he lost his gag reflex and his pupils don't respond when we shine a light in his eyes."

Ned fidgets in his chair. "In all honesty, I cannot continue to treat him like this. You have to understand that our treatments are demanding his body to work in impossible ways. We are torturing him with all our injections and blood draws." The staff nods their heads in agreement.

The Chen family does not show any emotional response to these words. Ned stops speaking for a few seconds. He looks around the room and says to the family, "My conscience demands that I switch him to comfort care. If I can't do that, then I'll have to sign off the case. We'll need to find you another doctor if you insist on continuing treatment. I will not be a part of this any longer."

Mrs. Wong hears his pain and lowers her voice. "Doctor, you must understand. I have no choice. Our culture demands that the eldest son makes these kinds of decisions. I know my father. This is what he would want. If he could talk, he would tell you that he wants his son to be here." Her sisters nod their heads in unison. "You must listen to me and honor our culture."

Ned responds, "I understand. You must take into account my solemn oath as a physician and the culture of intensive care. It demands that we do not inflict harm upon your father." His words rise in pitch and then stop.

Each side is certain their viewpoint is the right one and neither side is able to accept the other's position. My role is to assure that each view is heard and to initiate a compromise to satisfy Mr. Chen's family and the medical staff.

I swallow and take a quiet breath as I think of a possible solution. Mrs. Wong, "Are you certain your brother will be home by Monday?"

"Yes."

"In that case, will he be able to visit his father then?"

"Yes."

"Is it acceptable to you for the doctors to continue the current treatment without adding anything new?"

She looks at me. "Doctor, I have no problem with what is being done now. I just don't want anything stopped until Samuel gets here. If he dies before then, that would be fate and not our responsibility."

This is subtle, but important information. I immediately rephrase the compromise, spelling out exactly what it means for Mr. Chen's further care.

"Doctor Briggs, we've heard your concerns about continuing these treatments. In this light, will you continue Mr. Chen's current support until Monday? You wouldn't be expected to add any new therapy, even if he develops a complication like internal bleeding, another infection, or a major drop in blood pressure."

Ned answers with a deep sigh. "Reluctantly."

"Hopefully, Samuel will be here by then. If Mr. Chen doesn't show any signs of getting better by Monday, you'll initiate comfort care?"

Dr. Briggs nods his head and sighs.

"Mrs. Wong, your doctors told you that the current therapy would not reverse your father's dying process. He will not leave the hospital alive. You heard what the doctor said about further treatment going against his conscience, his own culture and that of the hospital. If he is no better over the weekend, the doctor will stop active treatment and move your father to comfort care even if your brother has not arrived. Can you accept that?"

"Yes, Doctor." She whispers as if she accepts her father's death is inevitable. Then continues, "If it is at all possible, our father would want Samuel to see him before the end comes."

"Mrs. Wong, it looks as if your father may not even make it through the weekend. I urge you to convey this information to your relative in Minnesota. Perhaps they can reach your brother before your father dies."

The conference was held Thursday afternoon. Mr. Chen quietly expired Friday evening. The nurses transferred his body from ICU to the hospital morgue because Mrs. Wong refused to release her father's body to the mortuary until Samuel arrived. Samuel came to the hospital Monday.

Reflections
Cultural Conflicts

The patients, physicians, and staff of a hospital community form a blend of cultures. Once it was unusual to hear a foreign tongue spoken in the hallways. Now, unfamiliar languages flowing throughout our medical centers often surround us.

A patient's ethnic background can affect his view of his ailment. He may ignore the physician's claim that bacteria or abnormal cancer cells are the cause of his illness. Instead, he may perceive God, fate, or the imbalance of human or body energy as the cause of his illness. Thus, he may refuse medical treatment. Home remedies and special rites may be more important to him than the use of pharmaceuticals or surgery.

Ethnicity plays a significant role in forming who we are, what we think, and how we act. It is a mistake to assume all peoples with the same background adhere to similar codes of ethics. Not all Hispanics live within a strong family unit. Not all American Indians accept the word of the tribe's shaman over that of the physician. Not all minorities of color fear white physicians who are directing their care. Not all white patients feel comfortable with physicians of color and/or gender.

Colliding beliefs and traditions can be a two way street. A patient's fear or mistrust of those with a different skin color, strange language, or the ways of Western medicine can be deep-rooted within his community and be difficult to change. The physicians and nurses are affected when a patient or family refuses to accept the staff's insistence that scientific treatment will benefit his well-being.

The staff must ask themselves what are the patient's beliefs and mores that they need to become aware of in order to understand their patient's reactions. This allows them to shape questions that aid in clarifying strongly held traditions and values and develop ways to work with their patient. Conversely, it is important for families to be made aware of the moral principles of the hospital and staff.

We can see how dilemmas develop when a patient and staff demand opposing actions to specific situations. The emotional trauma surrounding such a clash can be severe when each side insists that the other must ignore basic values that they hold dear. In Mr. Chen's situation, the conflict surrounding his family's ethnic mores concerning the status of the eldest son ignored the rapid deterioration of the father's condition.

When medical dilemmas occur, discussions between parties often deteriorate into polarization with each side standing firm as they tell their own *truths* without listening to other views. Autonomy[1] tells us to balance the values of the patient with those of the physician, staff, and hospital. Western medicine recognizes that conflicted decisions based on these standards should generally swing in favor of the patient. However, each person has an obligation to act according to her/his conscience.

With the Chen family, I wanted to create a free and protected space where each person could be heard with respect and with an open mind. I hoped that a compromise would be possible finding mutual agreement to what previously seemed insurmountable. Fortunately, Mrs. Wong was able to open a window that allowed her to save face. She would not be responsible for her father's death if he died receiving the present medical treatment. Dr. Briggs reluctantly agreed to wait for Mr. Chen's son to arrive in several days. They both accepted the continuation of the current regime without adding new treatment if complications occurred.

We can often nip a pending dilemma in the bud if care providers ask questions about themselves when facing similar situations that trigger a strong response:

- *What areas regarding this patient do I feel uncomfortable about and why?*
- *Where do I feel threatened, angry, or defensive?*
- *What helps me to reconsider the full body of facts, not just those that trigger my discomfort?*

Only when we know ourselves in these ways, we can choose to separate our issues from a presenting dilemma. Then we are free to approach our patient with compassion, concern, and curiosity. If we want to be an objective and creative advocate we must be willing to be present in a conflicting situation. We must let ourselves be *open to surprise.*

Our answer may surface from beneath a pile of discontent in unexpected ways. Movement can bring peace of mind to calm the frayed nerves of families and staff. It can be like a breath of fresh air flowing through an open window or a magnet discovering a pin in a haystack.

---

1. Chapter 1: *Living Life on the Edge* (Autonomy)
2. Chapter 11: *"I Love My Son"* (Case Conferences)

13

"Let Me Go!"

Hydration and Nutrition

Carol Reynolds is forty years old. She has a long history of a progressive neuromuscular disease. Five days ago, she attempted suicide by shooting herself in the mouth. The bullet fractured her cervical spine. Carol is now hemiplegic on her left side. She remains mentally clear. She refuses hydration, nutritional support, and further medical intervention other than pain control. Her husband requests an ethical conference to clarify the issues surrounding his wife's care.

I open an urgent email from Dottie Ferber, the nurse manager for the surgical unit: *Mike, please give me a call. We have a patient here who needs an ethics case conference as soon as possible.* I immediately pick up the phone.

"How can I help you, Dottie?"

"I appreciate your calling me back so quickly, Mike. My staff is in an uproar about this one. Although most of us are in agreement with the patient, some of my nurses think that doing what she wants would be repugnant as well as criminal. None of us are clear about what to do."

"Dottie, I hear that. I'm free right now. I'll come right over."

"Thanks, Mike. I'll be in my office."

I arrive at Dottie's office about ten minutes later. She is a lovely lady with a perpetual smile on her face. She motions me to sit down.

"My heart goes out to this lady and I want to do everything in my power to help her. Mike, I just don't know if it would be right to

97

follow her wishes. I worry that we'd be allowing her to commit suicide, or even helping to kill her."

"Whoa, you're going too fast. Please start at the beginning."

"Sorry." She unconsciously pulls at her ear. "Carol is in her forties and has had a neuromuscular disease for a long time. The disease has progressed enough that she has been bed-bound for the last six months. She now has difficulty swallowing and breathing."

An image of Stephen Hawking, one of my heroes, appears to me. He has been suffering from Amyotrophic Lateral Sclerosis (ALS) for a half-century. He continues to advance the field of theoretical physics with his magnificent mind. However, he is an exception. Most patients suffer immensely during the later stages of this disease. Carol is facing a similarly cruel death.

Dottie sighs, and continues. "She shot herself in the mouth a week ago when her husband was not home. She missed her brain but severed her spine. Now she is paralyzed on her left side and has severe neuropathic pain throughout her body."

"Oh, my God. That's awful. How on earth did she get ahold of a gun?"

"I don't know and I don't want to delve into that question. What is done is done." Dottie hesitates a moment and continues, "Her mind is clear as a bell and she insists she wants to stop eating and drinking. She wants us to control her pain and allow her to die."

"What does her husband say?"

"Well, he is in total agreement. He is asking for an ethics meeting to help clarify what can and should be done for his wife."

"She tried to commit suicide less than a week ago. Have you gotten a psychologist or psychiatrist to evaluate her mental status?"

"We got psych in yesterday. The doc says she's not depressed and has the capacity to make medical decisions for herself." Dottie swallows and wipes her forehead. "I don't know; it doesn't feel right."

"Let's set up a case conference. Help me make a list of the players who should be at there. Is she in a private room?"

"Yes."

"Great, let's meet at her bedside tomorrow afternoon at 1:00."

WE CAN, BUT SHOULD WE?

Fifteen representatives from a variety of therapies meet in Carol's room. They include Carol, her husband, several doctors, nurses, a social worker, her speech therapist, and the hospital chaplain. Each person present will hear and state various viewpoints.

Carol begins. She speaks slowly and with some difficulty because of her pain. However, she is clear as she repeats her insistence on stopping nutrition and hydration support. She describes her worsening condition. Her major concern is near total body pain. She puts it at a "100 on a scale of 0 to 10."

It is clear to all of us that Carol understands the dilemma she is in and the options available to her. We discuss the possibilities: continued palliative care in the hospital, rehabilitation in a skilled nursing facility, or home with hospice. Although a neurosurgical operation on her neck might ease her neuropathic pain, she refuses surgery. Carol's goal is for a comfortable death. Although she wants to have euthanasia, she knows that this is not yet legal in California.

This particular case brings up a number of emotionally charged issues for everyone who has contact with Carol. The psychiatrist tells us that even with her chronic disease and her failed suicide attempt she is capable of understanding the concept of the discontinuation of nutrition and hydration. He tells us that Carol is not depressed. She does have the capacity to make her own healthcare decisions. She understands that she is not actively dying, but, for Carol, her pain and disabilities are far worse than death. She wants to begin her dying process.

At first, this is a difficult concept for several members of the staff who feel that this type of care is a form of euthanasia. Medical ethics clearly shows that withholding of food and liquids is not euthanasia or murder when we justify this direction of care by showing its benefits outweigh its burdens from the patient's viewpoint. In addition it is not ethical to force-feed a patient against her will.

Following the conference, the staff meets in a nearby room to debrief. We all share our views regarding this issue. Eventually, everyone becomes comfortable with proceeding with Carol's wishes.

J. Michael Gospe, M.D.

Carol opts for palliation in the hospital and is transferred to the Palliative Care Unit five days after the conference. She receives intravenous opiates with only enough IV fluid to deliver the narcotics.

Carol dies several days later with her husband at her bedside.

Reflections
Hydration and Nutrition

The ethics of the delivery of hydration and nutritional support to a patient is in the same category as are all other medical interventions. The patient with capacity, or her surrogate, has the right to accept or reject medical treatment if the burdens outweigh the benefits of treatment *as seen from the patient's viewpoint.*

The question of the benefits and burdens of nutrition and hydration support is complex.[1,2] The goal of the healing professions is to prolong life and its quality. We learn techniques to reverse disease and repair damaged organs. When I was in my training fifty years ago, our instructors chastised and belittled us in front of our peers whenever a patient expired. I recall the *Death and Dying Rounds* when my Chief Resident would point a finger at one of us and infer fault. *Why did you let that happen? Didn't you know any better?* Little or no time was set aside to examine the goals of treatment from the patient's point of view. We never asked the sick person, *What is it you would like us to do for you?*

The balancing of benefits and burdens is easier to apply when surgery or medications are involved. When the withdrawal of hydration or nutrition becomes the focus, the situation becomes more complicated. The humane offering of food and water is a basic response entwined within our genes. I recall the chicken soup my Jewish grandmother gave me when I had a cold. After I was married, my wife's Italian mother came to our house with a pot of minestrone when our children were sick. Each knew their creation would nourish their loved one and provide healing.

With respect towards withholding nutrition or hydration, it is not uncommon for one to feel:

WE CAN, BUT SHOULD WE?

- *responsible for killing our patient or our loved one.*
- *negligent in giving their body the barest essentials to exist.*
- *passive that we are doing nothing but watching and waiting for the finality of our patient's death.*

We may imagine our loved one or patient shriveling up before our eyes, experience thirst as we moisten her mouth and lips, or feel hungry when the food cart passes her room. We must remember, when a patient is dying, her body's systems are shutting down, one by one. It is much like the airline pilot after he has landed his plane. He carefully switches off each of the many systems that had allowed the plane to soar towards the heavens with its cargo of passengers.

The withholding of fluid and nutrition does not create excessive thirst and hunger. As the patient dies, her brain, heart, lungs, and other systems weaken and begin to turn off. The intestinal tract cannot assimilate food at this point. Oral feeding often produces distention, diarrhea, abdominal pain, bloating, nausea, and vomiting. Further complications can ensue. The most common is pneumonia due to the aspiration of gastric contents. Nor can intravenous nutrition reverse a terminal process. It can allow for the possibility of the development of sepsis from resistant bacteria or fungi.

Carol's case was far different from the usual situation where physicians consider the withdrawal of hydration and nutrition. Carol was not actively dying. Rather, she wanted to avoid looking toward a prolonged, painful, and deteriorating slide toward death. With the exception of pain medication and comfort measures, she elected to refuse all medical treatment including nutrition and fluids. The dilemma for the staff was that the shutting down of her organs had not yet occurred. She was not in an acute dying mode.

The value of one's continued life is clearly personal. Generally, a physician, family member, or surrogate should not override it. From Carol Reynolds' viewpoint, she determined that prolonged straining to move or to breathe required additional drugs that created too great a burden on her body and her psyche. From her perspective, the burdens of her disease far outweighed the benefits of continued life. She had the right to refuse therapy and nutrition.

J. Michael Gospe, M.D.

On the other-hand, Stephen Hawking's productivity continues at an impressive rate as his illness takes its toll on his physical body. In his book, *A Brief History of Time*, Professor Hawking says:

> *Apart form being unlucky enough to get ALS, or motor neuron disease, I have been fortunate in almost every other respect. The help and support I received ... have made it possible for me to lead a fairly normal life and to have a successful career. I was again fortunate in that I chose theoretical physics, because that is all in the mind. So my disability has not been a serious handicap.*

Fortunately, the past quarter century has seen a change in the mindset of medical educators. Patient autonomy is now part of the equation when developing a care plan for an injured or sick person.[3] The balance between what we can do, what we should do, and what we will do is complex often requiring input from many sources. However, it remains difficult for all of us when we must watch a patient die at a time when we could institute technological steps to keep her alive.

At the same time, when intense emotions arise in the hospital setting, we must consider all of the participants as well as the patient. Identifying areas of anxiety and initiating a one-to-one discussion with the concerned patient, family, or staff member can often diffuse problems and create comfort where distress once existed. Any physician, nurse, or staff member who is unable to reconcile their beliefs with those of the patient regarding a specific form of therapy has the right to transfer off of a case if a replacement is available.

As long as our patient or surrogate has a truly informed consent about the potential consequences of the discontinuation of fluid and food and understands the risks and benefits of this decision, then it is morally justifiable to follow her wishes. When a patient or surrogate requests the medical profession to allow a natural death to occur, we change the emphasis of care from curative to comfort. I have often noticed a palpable sense of peace encircle the staff as they help the patient toward a more comfortable end of life when they follow their patient's lead.

WE CAN, BUT SHOULD WE?

1. Chapter 2: *Changing Image* (Beneficence)
2. Chapter 3: *Not a Leg to Stand On* (Non-Maleficence)
3. Chapter 1: *Living Live on the Edge* (Autonomy)

14
Out of the Box
Non-compliance

Craig Bartlett, a homeless double-amputee, is fifty-four years old. He suffers from dementia and chronic addiction to alcohol. He has been newly diagnosed with an HIV-AIDS infection. His past history reveals multiple hospitalizations for alcohol related problems and non-compliance with medical orders. The staff's concerns circle around the benefits and burdens of treatment options, post-hospital care, and available resources for his HIV disease.

I am sipping my second cup of coffee when I receive a phone call from Sam Payne, a physician in our hospital's Palliative Care Unit. He has been a member of my ethics committee for years. Sam only requests formal help with challenging cases that revolve around highly charged family issues or staff responses to end of life concerns.

In his relaxed and understated voice, Sam asks, "Mike, could you drop over to the unit this afternoon? I have a patient over here with a rather bizarre set of ethical problems."

My afternoon schedule looks light and I'm happy to get involved with a stimulating ethics encounter. "Sure, Sam, how about my coming over after lunch?"

"See you then."

I arrive at the unit at 12:30 and find him sitting at his desk. Sam, a slender man in his mid fifties, closes his computer when I arrive.

WE CAN, BUT SHOULD WE?

"Glad to see you, Mike. This situation is loaded with a bag of issues touching on almost every value in the book from individual autonomy, through benefits and burdens, and extending all the way to societal justice. On top of it all, my patient has a strong history of non-compliance and will probably put a monkey wrench into everything we try to do for him."

I feel my mind go into high gear and my juices begin to flow as I pull out a pen and piece of paper. "Start at the beginning."

"Mr. Bartlett lives near Railroad Square. A number of years ago, when the trains were still running, he passed out in a drunken stupor ending up sprawled-out over the tracks. An engine came by and amputated both of his legs."

"How in heck does he get around?"

"Believe it or not, he's very active in his wheel chair. He camps out in one of the parks near the tracks and eats at the Mission on Fifth Street." Sam groans a bit and continues. "I forgot to mention that he's a malnourished chronic alcoholic with a some early dementia. He also has Hepatitis B, Hepatitis C, chronic lung disease, and a seizure disorder." He swallows and adds, "The guy came to the hospital a week ago with one of his alcohol withdrawal seizures and pneumonia. Here is the main problem. One of the ER docs drew an HIV titer with his admission lab work. It came back yesterday strongly positive for HIV-AIDS."

"Does he have a family?"

"Nope. He severed all ties with everyone in his past."

"Whoops. And the ethical problem is?"

Sam looks at me and smiles, "Like the TV ads say, 'But there's more; just listen to this.'" He continues, "The guy has a long history of not keeping clinic appointments after each of his multiple admissions for pneumonias, seizures, and traumas." Sam becomes more serious, "The treatment for HIV-AIDS is pretty good now in 2008; we've come a long way in the past twenty or twenty-five years. My concern is that if we begin treatment and he doesn't follow through there's a good chance he'll develop a resistant strain of the virus. That could lead to a public health nightmare with super viruses infecting the community. On the other hand, if we don't start treatment, he'll die of AIDS."

105

"Have you thought about placing him in a convalescent facility while he is on treatment?"

"Won't work. He refuses to live anywhere other than on the streets. Besides, HIV treatment is for life."

"Boy, Sam, this is a tough one. Let's put together a meeting and see what we can come up with."

Sam and I develop a list of people with various backgrounds to help us form a viable plan of action for Mr. Bartlett. Ten of us meet; they include five physicians: Sam from Palliative Care; Rex, a hospitalist; Jeannie, an infectious disease specialist; Kent, the head of the local HIV clinic; and myself. A case manager, nurse, two lay representatives from an AIDS support group, and the hospital's Vice-President for Mission and Values are also present.

After Sam summarizes Mr. Bartlett's past and current history, we spend over an hour batting around the various treatment options available to us for in-hospital and post-hospital care.

I ask the group, "Anyone know exactly what his goals of treatment are?"

Rex responds, "Yeah. Mr. Bartlett keeps repeating that all he wants is to get back to his wheelchair and his camp in the park by the tracks." Rex shakes his head. "That will never happen. He doesn't understand the severity of his illness. The complications of his HIV are going to get worse. His ER and hospital visits will increase in frequency and severity until he finally dies."

Jeannie raises a question, "Is there any way we can find out how much of this man's mental problem is caused by alcohol and how much is due to HIV encephalopathy?"

Sam shrugs. "The only way we will ever know for sure is to treat him and see what happens."

Rex shares his frustration. "Bartlett has a grab bag of diagnoses, any one of them is bad, but the lot together is terrible."

"No kidding," Jeannie continues, "I'm amazed his pneumonia was easily controlled. He's darn lucky it wasn't a pneumocystis like we usually see with HIV secondary infections."

Sam adds, "Yeah, we can spiff him up and improve his nutrition. The thing that will kill him is the HIV. This other stuff is all chronic and can be relatively simple to handle." He looks toward Kent. "Kent, you've got much more experience with this virus than the rest of us put together. Is it ethical for us to offer him expensive and complex treatment? We know he won't comply with our medical regime and he is a candidate for inviting new strains of the bug."

"Look, everyone," Kent answers, "HIV is much easier to treat now compared to even only a couple of years ago. Luckily, the Feds cover all HIV medication and he is on MediCal. Funding won't be a problem. We have treatment available. We've got to treat him."

I feel we are beginning to spin our wheels. I look up from my notes and say, "Let's start with reviewing the benefits and burdens of all forms of treatment and non-treatment. First, what are the odds of resistant organisms showing up if he doesn't take his medication properly? If his past history means anything, he will probably fail his clinic visits from the outset."

"That's a biggie." Jeannie sighs, "I'm worried about the public health spin off. We don't want to get bad bugs into the community."

The rest of the group add their perspectives as we learn about the hospital's value of treating all patients, regardless of their mental, financial, or sociological condition. We hear about the options that the AIDS support group in the community has available for Mr. Bartlett. The nursing staff tells us how surprisingly easy it is for him to transfer to and from his wheelchair and get around the hospital corridors.

I look at the clock and scan the group. I see people are getting tired and we are reaching an impasse.

"It seems to boil down to whether or not he'll take his medications as an outpatient. If we can be reasonably assured that he will, then HIV treatment may be an option. If not, then we are back to palliative care until his HIV kills him." I continue, "Look, everyone, even though we have a big group here, I think we need some more input. What about starting HIV treatment to see if the encephalopathy gets better? Maybe that will improve his motivation to follow our course of treatment. Let's meet in a week or so and try to get the County Public Health Officer to join us. Seems to me that the risk of developing resistant organisms is too big to ignore. In the meantime, the social service folks at the HIV clinic can check their sources and see if any other agencies might be able to help. Now is the time for some out of the box thinking."

The group agrees with this plan and Mr. Bartlett starts treatment with retroviral agents in an attempt to bring down his HIV viral load.

About a week later, Mr. Bartlett leaves the hospital against medical advice. He is back in the ER within twenty-four hours after suffering another seizure. After another week, a Good Samaritan sees him in the park and calls an ambulance. Mr. Bartlett is confused and looks terrible. A mixture of feces and urine covers his body. He is dehydrated and his temperature is elevated. His physician begins intravenous antibiotics, fluids, and HIV medication.

The Public Health Officer joins the ten of us for our second meeting to discuss his situation.

Rex points out a fact that seems obvious to most of us in the room. "I'm now even more concerned about this guy's ability to successfully take all of his medicine as an outpatient."

Kent persists. "Yes, but I don't see anything to debate here. Your patient has a disease with effective treatment. Without treatment it will soon be lethal. We have extraordinary resources available to HIV patients in our clinic. Let's see if there is a way we can use these resources to help him."

The group continues to raise their concerns.

"Can he really give an informed consent for treatment? There aren't any relatives to speak for him."

"The guy's goal in life is to find his next cigarette and drink. Does he understand what is going on here?"

"Bartlett last left the hospital against medical advice where he had comfort, food, shelter, warmth, and medications. This was the best of all possible worlds for him. How on earth can we believe he will improve on his own?"

We spend a great deal of time mulling over the pros and cons of what to do. The Public Health Officer and the head of the HIV-AIDS clinic convince the rest of us to give him a one-month timed clinical trail of outpatient treatment. Kent comes up with a remarkable plan. The HIV clinic will purchase a global positioning unit to attach to his wheelchair. The clinic will then assign an outreach worker to track him down on a daily basis and see he takes all of his medications at one time each day.

I met one of the HIV physicians at a medical meeting five years later. I was both gratified and astounded to learn about Mr. Bartlett's response to this approach. After discharge from the hospital, he returned to his camp by the park. The outreach workers closely followed him for the next nine months. He showed steady improvement in his disease. His viral load eventually dropped to undetectable. During this time, the social worker discovered that Mr. Bartlett had an honorable discharge from the military and was eligible for a VA housing allowance as well as an in-home caregiver. Housing and care were located for him. He continued to thrive and had no emergency room visits in the last four years. His alcohol consumption dropped significantly although the mild dementia persisted. It appeared that he had gotten used to life in a warm room rather than out under the stars or fog of a cold night.

Reflections

Non-compliance

None of us who work in the hospital community are immune to the frustration that develops around the non-compliant patient. Over the years, I have had patients who refuse prescribed medications; won't allow dressing changes; or reject offered therapies. Even in my suburban hospital, we have patients whose friends sneak inappropriate food, tobacco, or street drugs into the hospital room. Others patients may deny access to case managers and social workers who are trying to identify insurance coverage, arrange for governmental aide, or establish post hospital care

Every case of non-compliance is unique. The difficult ones, such as we saw develop in Chapter 4, *The Shadow Side*, when Ms. Chapman interfered with her friend Dorothy Greenfield's care required persistence to arrive at a viable solution. Nursing and physician time is at a premium. It may seem far easier to bottle in our annoyance rather than to try to understand why the patient is acting that way. If we can change our mind set and accept the patient as the person he is, not the person we want him to be, then the rewards gained by *doing the right thing*[1] can be highly satisfying. This often may be achieved by taking a time out to have a one-on-one discussion with a colleague or chaplain. With complex cases, an administrative case conference might be preferable to help clear the air.

It became more problematical with Craig Bartlett. The staff knew from his past history that even if they were able to cure his current problem, he would soon return to the Emergency Room because of complications arising from his lifestyle. The staff often labels these people as *difficult patients*. Before long, an unannounced battle may develop between *we the staff* and *they the patient*.

The amount of time, energy, and cost to provide care under these circumstances expands as the patient's hospital stay lengthens. It is not easy to care for a patient who makes us *uncomfortable*. This was experienced in Chapter 15, *Inevitable Death*, with the staff and my relationship to Tony Grayson's wife and her expectations of a miracle.

These difficulties compound themselves

- if the staff takes a moral high road and says:
  - *He's not doing his part.*
  - *She won't let me care for her the way I know best.*

- or if the staff feels:
  - *Nothing I do makes any difference.*
  - *My heart isn't in it.*
  - *I don't want to work with this patient.*
  - *What good am I doing here?*

Members of the staff may want to withdraw care or may even fail to offer simple comfort when the patient resists all else. Eventually, the caregivers may give up trying and choose a path of least resistance. This is a clear setup for a classic lose-lose scenario. The patient receives what may be mediocre treatment as the staff finds themselves compromising their standard of care.

As in Mr. Craig Bartlett's case, I have found that the use of an administrative case conference[2] is extremely helpful in developing strategies to work in a more effective way. This type of meeting often invites creative planning when the cause of non-compliance comes to light: a result of illness, mental health/addiction, financial, or spiritual issues. A gathering of many minds with different professional experience can sometimes shed enough light on a seemingly insolvable situation. In turn, the staff receives direction and the energy to find a workable resolution to the dilemma.

The solution, as always, is to meet the patient where he or she is and to use appropriate and creative resources available whenever possible.

---

1. Chapter 17: *Further Reflections* (Dignity)
2. Chapter 11: *"I Love My Son"* (Case Conferences)

15
Inevitable Death
Miracles

Tony Grayson, a fifty-nine year-old man, has been in the hospital for three weeks with severe peripheral vascular disease and multi-system failure. He is disorientated and cannot speak for himself. His wife waits for a miracle of healing. She insists on active treatment and full resuscitation if he were to experience a cardiac arrest. The staff observes that Mr. Grayson is actively dying and that changing his therapy to comfort care is appropriate.

My cell phone rings as I walk down Doyle Park Drive, a tree-lined residential street near the hospital. Walking clears my mind as I take in the spring colors that shout for attention in the nearby gardens.

Jeffery Adams is on the phone. He is a palliative care physician who sits on the hospital's ethics committee with me.

"Hi, Jeff. What's up?"

"I have just seen a man in ICU North; his name is Tony Grayson. It's clear he's going to die very soon. The intensive care doc and the surgeon have done all that they can and have asked me to help them switch their goals to comfort care rather than curative ones. The problem is that the man's wife insists that a miracle will occur and demands that the physicians continue to go all out with every medicine in the book."

"What is he on now?"

WE CAN, BUT SHOULD WE?

"He's been receiving tube feedings and is on a ventilator as well as a combination of cardiac medications, antibiotics, and fluids. He hasn't responded to any of these treatments during the past three or four days. Mike, this is terribly frustrating for the nurses and docs, including myself. Everyone feels that they're beating him with a *cat o' nine tails*."

I turn around and head back to the hospital. "I am only a block away. I'll pop back to the ICU and have a look at him. I'll call you when I'm done."

"Thanks, Mike. The staff will be grateful for anything you can do to help defuse the situation."

I enter the unit. All of the beds are filled with patients attached to beeping monitors and flashing screens. The whiteboard confirms that Tony Grayson is in room 241.

Inside his room, Mr. Grayson, a deeply jaundiced and cachectic man, lies in a coma. His abdomen forms a dome that is most likely filled with ascitic fluid. His cardiac monitor shows he is experiencing rapid atrial fibrillation. His blood pressure and central venous pressures are low and his respiratory rate rapid. Two IV's drip fluid into his veins. I notice rosary beads and a small cross on his bedside table. I say a silent prayer as I look at his chart at the nurses' station.

Mr. Grayson appears far older than his fifty-nine years. His body shows signs of chronic alcohol liver disease superimposed with a Hepatitis C infection. These conditions have resulted in the accumulation of ascitic fluid in his abdomen; gastrointestinal bleeding from his esophagus; seizures; malnutrition; and confusion. Added to that, he has severe ischemia of the right leg even after multiple surgical procedures: toes on both of his feet are at risk of becoming gangrenous. In addition, he suffers from acute respiratory failure from pneumonia, heart failure, and fluid in his pleural cavity.

At the present moment, mechanical ventilation keeps his blood oxygen at a reasonable level. Even so, coronary artery disease and persistent atrial fibrillation compromise his heart. He is in shock with a very low blood pressure.

Further scanning of the chart shows that several physicians have discussed Mr. Grayson's serious condition with his wife. She insists that there will be a miracle. She wants the doctors to continue full therapy. From what I see in the chart, I believe it is a miracle he is alive.

I schedule a case conference for 10:30 the next morning. The social worker invites Mrs. Grayson and suggests she bring family members for support. The intensive care physician, a hospital chaplain, and another member of the ethics committee will join Jeff and me at the meeting.

The staff arrives promptly at 10:30. Mrs. Grayson is yet to be seen by 10:45 so some members of the hospital team leave to attend to other matters. I am about to go at 11:00 when she arrives accompanied by several members of her family and a priest.

Mrs. Grayson is a petite woman with a gentle demeanor. I am surprised when she speaks with a commanding voice as she announces, without an excuse or apology for her delay, "There will be no meeting until my son arrives. He will be here in five minutes."

I swallow my discomfort and take her at her word. I call the ICU and ask a nurse to contact the other members of our team to see if they will be able to return to the conference room. With the exception of the intensive care physician and social worker, the staff reassembles.

Over the next few minutes, we are joined by seven members of the Grayson family and their pastor. Mrs. Grayson continues to insist that her son will arrive shortly. The minutes tick by. Her son finally arrives at 11:30. Mrs. Grayson says, "Now we can begin."

I attempt to hide my anger, take a deep breath, and begin the meeting by inviting each person to introduce his/herself. Unfortunately, my discontent with the family continues as I notice repetitive pacing, exiting, and reappearing of one or another of our guests during the next hour. To make matters worse, several members of the family have frequent outbursts with raised voices and crying spells.

Mrs. Grayson stands up and looks directly at each of us in the small room. Her relatives nod their heads in unison when she insists, "We expect a miracle to occur and you better not stop doing everything until God heals him. I do not want anyone speaking about death in my husband's room. He is not dying!"

WE CAN, BUT SHOULD WE?

At this point, I turn to Jeff and ask him to speak. He speaks to the family with concern as he presents the facts simply. "Unfortunately, there are no medicines that can reverse your husband's decline." He goes on to suggest comfort care. "We will use pain medication and sedatives so he will be comfortable to the end."

I observe Mrs. Grayson's stony silence before I ask their pastor, Father Lewis, to add words of solace for us all.

Father Lewis is a thin man in his late sixties dressed in black with a white collar. I see him pull out a rosary from his pocket and finger the beads as he tells his story.

"I was assigned to a church in New Mexico several years ago where I attended a ninety-two year-old lady who was dying. The doctors believed she would die within a matter of hours or days. I prayed at her bedside, not realizing she did not speak English and could not understand me. Nonetheless, the next day she improved. The doctors discharged her later that week. She lived another two years. This was a miracle. I am certain there will be one for Mr. Grayson. He will live!"

I am not prepared for his story. With each word, Father Lewis adds more sticks onto the smoldering fire around us. There is a palpable heaviness in the room. I notice the caregiver team squirming in their seats. My heart sinks into my chest. The moments crawl by. I hope the words will come soon.

The staff's respect for the Grayson value system and belief in miracles is in direct conflict with the staff's knowledge of Mr. Grayson's impending death and our desire to keep him comfortable at all cost. The family's demands allow no room for discussion.

Then Jeff catches my eye and nods to me. He restates his deep concerns about Mr. Grayson's inability to survive much longer. He adds, "Everything we are doing will not reverse Mr. Grayson's dying process. If his heart stops and we attempt to restart it, his ribs will break and the electrical shocks will burn his chest, causing him to suffer. He will die in extreme pain."

Jeff takes a breath here before proclaiming, "In good conscience, I must stop treatments that are not working. First, I will write a No Code order in his chart so there will be no attempts at CPR, which will do harm to his weakened body." He looks directly at Mrs.

Grayson when he says, "I am going to shift to comfort care, titrate down the blood pressure medicines, and stop all other unnecessary treatments like the antibiotics." His eyes scan the room, momentarily stopping on each member of the Grayson family. "I promise, we will do everything in our power to keep him comfortable."

He focuses on Fr. Lewis when he adds, "We will watch for any sign of improvement. Continue to pray for a miracle. When one occurs, we will certainly reevaluate our plans. In the meantime, I encourage you to use this time to support each other and say your goodbyes."

Mrs. Grayson shakes her head. "The family and I are the only people with the right to discontinue his ventilator."

There will be no compromise. A veil of fatigue glazes over our eyes. It was a long hour for the twelve of us in that airless room to hold our bodies and mind taut.

Jeff's approach is reasonable, ethical, and respective of Mr. Grayson's suffering. He agrees to continue mechanical ventilators at the family's strong request but will otherwise do what he can to make his patient more comfortable.

The Staff tapers down the medications. Mr. Grayson expires later that day. The family and their priest pray at his bedside until his last breath.

Reflections
Miracles

The Merriam-Webster Dictionary defines a miracle to be *an unusual or wonderful event believed caused by the power of God.*

It is not unusual for a conflict to arise between a patient's family and the healthcare staff when the family's faith assures them that God will heal their loved one and the staff is aware of the patient's dismal prognosis as his body shuts down. This can create discomfort, disagreement, mistrust, and eventual hostility. The ability to gently approach this type of situation with compassion is a skill learned by experience.

WE CAN, BUT SHOULD WE?

We each come to our death and the death of our loved ones in our own way. In my career, I have been fortunate to witness many of what I call *good* deaths. These are deaths that occur when patients and their families accept the fact that dying is happening. When the patient and family embrace the dying process, there is far less suffering for everyone. In fact, it is possible for the family to come together as one body even as they remain diverse in their grieving. I have been honored to be present and to be graced during this sacred time of ending.

The time when a patient's family cannot accept that the patient is dying before their eyes, I call a *bad* death. I have witnessed anger and denial grow to the point where the family remains blinded to their dear one as he ebbs away in their midst.

As we saw in this chapter, Mr. Grayson's body suggested a limited life span. His family's vision of a miraculous healing kept them from noticing that he was failing and would soon die. At the same time, the staff was intimately aware that he was dying. They found it difficult to say that they were unable to reverse his worsening condition. Yet, they knew the addition of more medicines would increase suffering only to prolong the inevitable.

In these circumstances, it is the job of healthcare providers to evaluate the benefits and burdens of prescribed treatments and therapies and to provide that critical information to the family in a way that the family could understand. From the staff's point of view, a switch in their goal of therapy from *curative* to *comfort* allows them to simplify his regime by discontinuing daily weights, blood tests, and numerous medications that now offer no chance of improving his deteriorating condition. Instead, they can concentrate on controlling his pain and anxiety while they allow his friends and family to remain at his beside to offer their love and support.

As in Mr. Grayson's situation, his family did not understand how this could be true. They misconstrued *comfort care* as meaning *no care*. In their minds, doing nothing left no room for hope. This could have been their first experience of being with a loved one who was mortally ill. A sea of emotions blurred their ability to integrate the confusing medical information that the healthcare team attempted to share with them. They remained confident that their loved one would arise from sleep against all odds.

The Grayson family's focus blocked them from changing to a course that they interpreted would *cause* him to die. This would be a decision that they knew would show their God they lacked faith. As long as Tony Grayson was alive under any circumstances, he was available for a miraculous healing.

The staff was also experiencing moral stress. They knew Mr. Grayson had little time left. They interpreted a plea for supernatural healing as a form of denial or an unrealistic coping mechanism. It was difficult for them to accept the importance of the family's belief system.

When dealing with a situation like this, it is not helpful for the staff to say:

- *If God wanted a miracle, then He would make one without the need for medications and a respirator.*
- *Perhaps the miracle is that God is giving you time to say your goodbyes.*
- *Perhaps the miracle is your coming together as one during this difficult time.*

Those words do not speak to the fear Mrs. Grayson was experiencing about how *giving up* would be her *responsibility*. Worse yet, these statements would belittle her religious beliefs.

In the midst of a dilemma, a listening ear by a hospital chaplain or a clergy member can sometimes provide a crack in the wall of denial. Sitting with the patient and/or family in periods of silence or openness goes a long way toward creating caring and compassion. Tears often signal a softening of one's immovable stance. Unfortunately, in Mr. Grayson's case, his pastor's lack of a medical background and his experience in New Mexico was not a helpful way to open a grieving place for Mrs. Grayson.

The art of active listening[1] by each member of the team can often help break an impasse. During the case conference, Jeff's words offered a compromise that he could accept and gave heed to one of the family's wishes as well. At the same time he refused to offer futile treatment that went against medical standards of care.

On the other hand, if Mr. Grayson had been alert, had an informed consent, and wished to continue standard care based on his *own*[2] goals, then the staff would have honored his wishes even as they knew he was soon to die.

A compassionate caregiver can offer a sincere attitude while giving care, hoping that the family will come to accept the patient's dire condition.

---

1. Chapter 17: *Further Reflections* (Active Listening)
2. Chapter 1: *Living Life on the Edge:* (Autonomy)

16
Home?
Access to Care

Jackson Cook is a forty-eight year-old homeless quadriplegic who has been in our acute care hospital for three years. Case Management has not been able to locate appropriate long-term care for him. The staff realizes Mr. Cook is using the hospital as his personal rehabilitation facility. They ask for a repeat conference to review and create new placement possibilities.

I pick up the phone on its third ring hearing a familiar voice on the line. "Is Dr. Gospe there?"

"Speaking."

"Hi, Doctor. This is Thelma, the case manager on Palliative Care. I called to see if you'd be available for a conference tomorrow afternoon at 2:30."

"Good to hear your voice. I'm checking my calendar as we speak. Ah, yes, I'm free at that time. What's up?"

"It's about Jackson Cook. I'd like to set up another administrative conference to see if anyone has new ideas on how we can transfer him to a more appropriate facility."

It takes a moment for me to recall Mr. Cook. Then his image comes through bright and clear. Mr. Cook is a quadriplegic with wasted muscles and extensive skin breakdown. I remember his body being covered with dressings when I saw him four or five months ago. His neurological disease and previous lifestyle have aged him beyond his forty-eight years. "I thought he'd been released by now."

120

WE CAN, BUT SHOULD WE?

"Unfortunately, we're still stymied about where to place him. I'm hoping you'll add something we haven't thought of."

After the call, I pull out my old notes on Mr. Cook. With a fresh piece of paper and my trusty pen in hand, I review my records and boot up his electronic medical record on my computer. There are extensive history, consultation, and physician notes from his admission in April 2001 to the latest summary dated February 2004. Upon reviewing them, I am able to fill in the details of his unique story.

Twenty-seven years ago, in 1977, Mr. Cook was a passenger riding in the back seat of a friend's car. The car collided with another automobile. A heavy object struck him on the back of his head, injuring his cervical spine. This accident left him without the use of his hands, legs, and feet. He does retain slight use of his arms.

During the years following his injury, he developed multiple decubitus ulcers on his body that required constant wound care treatment both in the hospital and various local skilled nursing facilities.

This current admission began three years ago. Infections of deep ulcerations on both of his legs and most of his gluteal area precipitated sepsis and shock. He required a colectomy to divert his stool from open wounds because of constant fecal soiling. He has a permanent urinary catheter placed through his abdominal wall so his urine will not further irritate his skin. The doctors are certain that his skin ulcerations will require intermittent intensive care and treatment for the rest of his life. After a month of stabilization in the surgical unit, his physicians transferred Mr. Cook to a bed in our Palliative Care Unit.

Mr. Cook has no family. Following his accident, he lived in various motels, on the streets, in different hospitals, and in jail. This current hospital stay is the longest time he has lived in the same place for many years.

I enter the Palliative Care Unit to have a look at Mr. Cook. The building is across the street from the hospital and was developed for patients during the terminal stages in their diseases. I am impressed by the comfort in these rooms; they are a far cry from those in the hospital. Each room is set up as a bedroom for a single patient and contains bedside tables, soft chairs, and brightly painted walls. A large library for patients and their families sits at one end of the building. A dining hall for ambulatory patients is at the opposite end.

Jackson Cook lies in bed watching a talk show on a television attached to the wall. He is an alert African-American man who speaks with a quiet voice and appears somewhat withdrawn. When he opens his mouth, I am immediately aware of his poor teeth. Some are decayed, some broken, and some missing. He wears a blue hospital gown that barely covers extensive dressings over his sacrum, legs, feet, and thighs. A functioning colostomy bag and a urinary tube draining fluid are located on his abdomen.

Even though he has paralyzed hands and legs, he has enough use of his arms to gradually pull himself up in bed. He tells me, "My skin ulcers are a lot better. So is my strength." He adds, "I'm now able to transfer myself to a wheelchair from bed."

I pull up an easy chair next to his bed, look at him, and continue our conversation. "What medical treatments are you getting now?"

"The nurses change my dressings every day or two and I see the wound care specialist now and then. My depression left me a few months ago. I'm on a bunch of pills and the pain patch keeps the pain way down." He smiles as he relates, "On Sundays people from the church come and take me to services."

I quietly shake my head in amazement when he continues, "Last summer I was able to visit the Sonoma County Fair with some nurses. In September they took me to Guerneville to the Russian River Jazz Festival. I really like it here in the hospital. I hope they won't be able to find a SNF (Skilled Nursing Facility) for me somewhere else. This is a great place to live."

I can see why the staff is frustrated. They see their hospital turned into a boarding house for Mr. Cook.

The next day, a group of doctors, nurses, social workers, and case managers meet in the Palliative Care Unit library for an administrative case conference. We brainstorm ideas that might help us determine a place where Mr. Cook can receive a more appropriate level of care.

122

WE CAN, BUT SHOULD WE?

Although Mr. Cook is comfortable in his current surroundings and is willing to stay as a patient in the unit for the rest of his life, it is clear to all of us that an indefinite continuation of the status quo is not an appropriate use of a hospital bed. There are sicker patients who require the services that he is receiving and our patient no longer requires skilled nursing care. Of more importance, our unit does not maintain Mr. Cook's dignity as an independent human being and it is not in his emotional or social interest to remain here for the rest of his life.

Trudy, the manager of our Case Management Department, summarizes the factual situation beautifully. "There are a number of reasons why a SNF will not consider accepting Mr. Cook as a patient. He is on MediCal. His lack of a work history denies him eligibility for Medicare.

Mr. Cook's wounds require extra nursing time and his quadriplegia necessitates he receive assistance with everyday functions. These needs, combined with his low-grade depression, some behavioral issues, and his young age would require a social activity program wherever he went. He would fill a long-term bed without the possibility of turnover. SNFs prefer patients who do not stay for years."

A nurse looks at Trudy and comments, "The bottom line is that he is truly at a SNF's level of care, but his needs far outweigh the payment any facility will receive from MediCal."

One of the doctors asks, "Is it possible for the hospital to pay for the extra care that would not ordinarily be provided by MediCal?"

Trudy answers, "That might be illegal. Generally, the State does not allow us to supplement MediCal's payments, but it's a reasonable idea. I will look into it with our legal people."

We toss around other ideas. Our group thinks that the idea of trying to augment a SNF's costs could be an effective way to move Mr. Cook to a more appropriate level of care.

Trudy contacts the legal and compliance officer for our health system. For this unique situation, the compliance officer arranges with the State to allow the hospital to pay for Mr. Cook's charges for any skilled assistance not covered under MediCal. Trudy's staff locates a specialized board and care facility in another county willing to accept

123

him under this waiver. This plan will be in effect for a specific period of time or until he becomes an inpatient at another hospital.

I have not been able to obtain any information concerning Mr. Cook since his discharge from our hospital.

Reflections

Access to Care

Charles Dickens in *A Tale of Two Cities* could have been writing about the American healthcare system in the early Twenty-first Century when he wrote *It was the best of times, it was the worst of times, it was the age of wisdom, it was the age of foolishness, it was the epoch of belief, it was the epoch of incredulity...*[1]

We have a powerful healthcare system in our country with state of the art medications, treatments, hospitals, and providers of care for those with health insurance or disposable funds.

However, we also have a large disenfranchised population who either cannot afford or cannot gain access to care as a result of a frayed medical safety net. Even with the Affordable Care Act, every one of us can tell stories of patients who face one or more barriers that make it difficult or impossible for them to receive adequate medical care.

Mr. Cook was comfortable in our hospital setting; it met most of his needs. However, his prolonged stay at our hospital was a triple-edged sword. It kept him from social interactions in a community. It affected the nursing staff when a patient needed a bed in the Palliative Care Unit, but were prevented admission because of a lack of beds. Finally, the institution's financial status was at risk because the payments from MediCal were well below the cost of Mr. Cook's care in an acute hospital.

The value of justice demands that we should try to be as fair as possible when offering treatment to a specific patient when allocating scarce medical resources. This requires evaluating the narrow tightrope that bridges what is best for our patient and what is available. In Mr. Cook's situation the lack of sufficient community resources made it impossible to find him long-term placement.

This dilemma reminds me of Freshman Orientation Camp at Caltech. The Dean of Students made a comment to my fellow students that I have never forgotten. *We know you are all intelligent; otherwise, we would not have accepted you to our school. What we expect to teach you the next few years is how to be aware of what it is you do not know and where to locate the correct answers.*

I have tried to live my life following his words of wisdom by not being afraid to reach out and ask for advice from those with a different yet complimentary expertise than mine. Faced with an insoluble problem as in Mr. Cook's complicated case, I encouraged tapping the expertise of people within our hospital as well as organizations within the community. I invited them to join in multidisciplinary conferences concerning our patient[2] in the hopes they would offer new approaches to our dilemma.

Here are several important things for all of us to ponder:

- *What are we most concerned about?*
- *What don't we know?*
- *What questions should we ask?*
- *How or where can we find our answers?*

When involved with a medical dilemma of limited resources, it is helpful to pay attention to the one or two steps in front of you, not the overall marathon. As with Mr. Cook, we found a timely but limited solution.

When physicians and family are considering problems regarding access to care, here are some life-style difficulties to be aware of:

- *The lack of adequate transportation to medical offices, clinics, and hospitals.*
- *The scarcity of primary care physicians located in his disadvantaged community.*
- *The differences in language and culture between his healthcare providers and himself.*

Or, as with Mr. Cook, the problem may revolve around:

- *The lack of needed psychiatric care.*

J. Michael Gospe, M.D.

- *The shortage of durable medical medications and equipment.*
- *Hospital beds needed for sicker patients.*
- *Social needs for his specific situation.*

Even if our country had universal healthcare insurance, we would still find it difficult to determine the appropriateness of using limited resources for our patients. On occasion we may find ourselves withdrawing needed care or even failing to offer it in the first place. This is not a theoretical problem. Even today, it is not unusual to have a limited supply of opioids for pain relief, chemotherapeutic medications for cancer treatment, sera for immunizations, or antibiotics for dangerous infections.

Every case is unique. The difficult ones require a significant amount of time and energy to evaluate and arrive at a viable solution. In difficult situations such as the one the staff faced with Mr. Cook, the giving everyone permission to reach *out of the box*[3] for answers, resulted in a win-win for the patient, staff, and hospital. All of our time is at a premium and its use can be costly. We must never forget that an elusive answer often comes only after intense searching.

---

1. Dickens, Charles. *A Tale of Two Cities.* Bantam Classic. 1983. Pg.1
2. Chapter 11: *"I Love My Son"* (Case Conferences)
3. Chapter 14: *"Out of the Box"* (Non-compliance)

17
Further Reflections
Dignity, Informed Consent, Active Listening

As seen in the previous chapters, a constellation of causes produces heart-rending conflicts between patients, families, and hospital staff. Some issues smolder for days or weeks like Dorothy Greenfield's situation in Chapter 4, *The Shadow Side,* where Ms. Chapman gradually inserted herself in her friend's care in ways that an atmosphere of mistrust gradually brewed between the staff and patient/friend.

Others can flare into supernovae overnight and cause havoc before anyone is aware of their existence as with Carol Juleps in Chapter 2, *Changing Image,* when, in a rare moment of clarity, Carol decided to have her legs amputated.

The truth is that all of us are called to be ethicists when it comes to issues related to life and death. We are all alive until we reach that unyielding finish line called death. Every step of the way on our journey contains an infinite number of hurdles. Many of them seem to be insurmountable as the prospect of death draws ever nearer. Our instilled values, our spiritual essence, and our previous experiences all play a part in how we deal with the end of our life or the dying of a loved one. Caregivers and family should never forget to place our patient first as he continues his final earthly journey.

It is important that the hospital staff not assume what their patient and the patient's family are feeling when under pressure. Conversely, the patient and family may not comprehend the reasons for specific medical treatment; in fact, they may deem them inappropriate or just plain wrong. Time for providing opportunities for inclusive communication is key to reaching a peaceful end. An opening of minds and hearts for all can evolve when everyone can listen to each other.

This chapter will discuss three further topics that can affect the solving of ethical dilemmas: Dignity, Informed Consent, and Active Listening.

Dignity

A specific set of values lies at the heart of medical ethics in Western medicine. The hospital where I serve as the Director of Medical Ethics espouses four values for all members of their staff to follow: Dignity, Service, Excellence, and Justice. To my mind, dignity of a human being is fundamental to all of these. Our hospital defines dignity as *respecting each person as an inherently valuable member of the human community and as a unique expression of life.*

Loss of dignity comes in many forms such as:

- cold meals sitting on the bedside table or in front of patient who is too weak to feed herself.
- bed covers lying bunched up at the side of the bed, exposing the patient's thinly clad body.
- the patient's glasses or hearing aides lying unused in a drawer.

In these situations and many others, it is the family's obligation to bring this information to the staff. It is the caregiver's responsibility to honor the patient's desires and to address any problems that lead to a loss of her dignity.

The value of dignity encompasses:

- *Autonomy*[1]: the patient has the right to control the breadth and length of her care.
- *Beneficence*[2]: the primary caregiver is obliged to do what is helpful for his patient, to compare benefits and burdens of all treatment options *from the patient's point of view*, and to emphasize those actions that aide his patient.

WE CAN, BUT SHOULD WE?

- *Non-maleficence*[3]: the caregiver should lean in the direction of not harming his patient or going against her wishes.
- *Justice*[4]: although the patient comes first, it is important for the caregiver to treat his patient and the rest of society as fairly as possible, especially in the face of scarce medical resources.
- *Fidelity*[5]: the caregiver should answer questions regarding the patient's diagnosis, prognosis, and treatment with compassion and truth.

This current value of dignity is in contrast to how medicine was practiced in the mid Twentieth Century where the patient was kept in the dark. At that time, Western Medicine stood on a pyramidal or patriarchal platform. The physician perched high at the apex while the patient and her support community remained far down at the base with the rest of the staff somewhere in between. The attending doctor, thought to be the expert on all things concerning medicine and treatment options, made all of the decisions.

In the late nineteen-fifties when I was in college, my grandmother was dying of metastatic carcinoma of the colon. My physician father and his colleagues elected not to inform her of her condition or prognosis. They believed that if she knew these facts, she would not want to live. Because I was in college at that time, my parents shielded me from this situation until I returned home for summer vacation. Though I now understand their reasoning, I still mourn that I did not have a chance to say *Goodbye* to her.

Twenty years later, when I was in the early years of my practice of gastroenterology, the concept of patient autonomy had not changed from the time of my grandmother's death. For example, I was not mentored to explain all of the risks of a colonoscopy to my patients. I thought, along with my colleagues, that they would become frightened and refuse the needed intervention.

The past three decades have seen a major change in medical ethics. Now, we bring our patients into the decision loop early. We ask that they become aware of all treatment options, their risks and benefits. The patient is at the top of the triangle here. It is the caregiver's responsibility to honor his patient's desires.

The value of dignity also applies to the healthcare provider. A physician, nurse, or other staff member is never under an ethical obligation to offer any treatment that is contrary to the accepted standard of care in the community or that is incompatible with his or her own moral code. If a caregiver feels it necessary to leave a case, he or she is obligated to tell this to the patient and family and to find trained personnel to take over the care of the patient.

Informed Consent

Today, it is illegal to perform a medical procedure on a patient with capacity without obtaining an informed consent. For the physician to not comply is considered to be a form of legal battery upon the patient. An informed consent allows our patient to better choose her treatment from among alternatives. This allows her to contribute and participate in her care. She is part of the care team, not just a body or a disease in a designated room.

If a patient does not have capacity, the physician has a duty to locate an appropriate surrogate decision-maker to give permission for treatment.[6,7] In urgent situations, one or two physicians may sign the consent. In non-urgent situations, the hospital's social worker, bioethics consultant, or risk manager can help find a suitable person to help make these decisions.

The physician's role in obtaining approval to perform a procedure or to begin or stop treatment must fulfill several obligations. He is required to know that the patient:

- *Understands* the regimen's options, major benefits, and burdens in simple terms.
- *Appreciates* the benefits and the risks of different proposed treatments or no treatment at all.
- *Reasons* and sifts through medical information and relates this information to her personal values.
- *Communicates* back to her physician how and why she has made her decision.

WE CAN, BUT SHOULD WE?

A *complete* informed consent is frequently not obtained. It is not uncommon for a consent discussion to lack all necessary information. For example, when asked to consent for the performance of CPR in the case of a cardiac arrest, the physician may have asked, *Do you want us to do everything we can to keep you alive?* Nowhere in the conversation was any mention made concerning the success or failure rate of CPR performed in patients with a similar age and disease, the probable occurrence of broken ribs, painful shocks, and intubation, nor information regarding the patient's ability to return to a baseline level of function.

Even when statistics are mentioned, they are often not made clear to the patient. In comparing treatment option A with option B, the patient may hear that the newer medication results in patients living twice as long than with the older medication. The facts that this extension of life may be from two weeks to six months and would likely result in multiple side effects and marked suffering at a cost of thousands of dollars of future care are omitted.

Over the years as both a physician and a patient, I have discovered that the best way to be certain that needed information is obtained is when the patient makes a list of the questions they want answered by the physician and brings that list, preferably with a relative or friend, to the doctor's appointment. All too often, when the "C" word is mentioned, the patient tends to block out further information that the doctor has to tell her. Looking for answers on the Internet is a mistake that most of us, including myself, make when we bypass our own physician and go searching for answers on our own. It is best to seek out an expert second opinion.

Obtaining a truly informed consent demands that patients hear the whole truth and are *given time* to consider the options set before them.

Active Listening

When you talk, you are only repeating what you already know
If you listen, you may learn something new
Dali Lama

J. Michael Gospe, M.D.

Although this section is written primarily to help physicians and staff who may be involved in complex multidisciplinary patient care conferences, its information can be quite helpful for patients and families who find it difficult to communicate with each other and with the hospital's physicians and staff.

Active listening is an art. It is more than just sitting with a patient or family member, asking questions, and listening to the answers. It is:

- *making* eye contact.
- *being curious.*
- *having* open posture.
- *putting aside* assumptions and agendas.
- *being open* to allow new information to surface.
- *inviting* everyone to unpack their questions and concerns in a non-judgmental atmosphere.

Active listening is a learned skill that allows a dialogue between *equals* rather than participating in several monologues wrapped around each other; often with one asserting more power over another. When people feel listened to, it is easier for hidden stories to come to light. These experiences can reveal the reasons for strongly held views that color one's perception.

Unfortunately, it is common for a physician, staff member, or patient's family to lose objectivity and project his or her experience or knowledge onto that of the patient. The active listening process during Clyde Anderson's case conference in Chapter 1, *Living Life on the Edge* allowed the staff and myself to change our viewpoints concerning his care after we had the opportunity to hear about his life with Mrs. Anderson and with his motorcycle friends. In Fred Franklin's case conference in Chapter 11, *I Love My Son,* Fred's wife Joan shared a memory of conversations the two had concerning their own wishes while she was writing a term paper about end of life decisions. This changed everything. It was if Fred was speaking directly to his mother and sister. This released their burdens as they were now able to understand his own wishes concerning the care he would likely want.

WE CAN, BUT SHOULD WE?

We caregivers must remember that this may be the first time that our patients and their family have faced a life threatening disease. They may not be able to conceive or understand the rapidity of the disease process. They may be overwhelmed by thoughts of the eventual outcome, pain, suffering, financial effect, and change that will affect all of their lives in the future. Acute stress surrounding a loved one's illness often clouds their ability to listen clearly and to express their viewpoints to others in the family and to the healthcare team. They may be fixated on inadequate and outdated information or myths regarding treatment. They may be afraid or feel incompetent to ask questions as they carefully watch caregivers hoping to glean some knowledge about what is happening as busy nursing personnel and physicians read the latest data on monitors, smile, and leave the room without interacting with the visitor.

Those of us who work in hospital settings follow seriously ill patients on a daily basis. We must be mindful of how we express ourselves to our patient and his family. With each encounter, it is wise to ask ourselves:

- *Am I automatic and curt?*
- *Do I meet them eye-to-eye, smile, and offer them kind words?*

When faced with a medical dilemma, it is important to find the time and make the opportunity for dialogue and active listening. These are necessary components for describing the patient's current status and airing misconceptions head on, before they become polarizing.

There are several simple but very effective active listening techniques that we can use at the bedside or in a group setting.

- *Rephrase* statements in a way that will help clarify what others are saying. This ensures that they have been heard correctly.
- *Be aware* of body language and alert to hidden messages such as fear, anxiety, or disagreement.

133

- Make *simple statements* that may give that person permission to talk.
    - *I see you are uncomfortable. Would you like to add something?*
- *Keep in mind* that extroverts tend to think out loud whereas introverts often need time to think before they speak and may need an invitation to participate.

Physicians and staff members also need to remember to:
- Be *gentle,* kind, listen carefully, ask for clarity when needed.
- Be *straightforward,* listen to concerns, watch body language for clues.
- Be *factual* and then *wait* for a response.
- Offer a *recommendation.*
- Give a *choice.*
- *Highlight* the important facts, be certain the patient understands.

A formal case conference[8] that uses the technique of active listening can help update and clarify medical aspects, air concerns and ease conflict or confusion. These meetings are not about *dictating* a path for another's life or death. Instead, they are about *defining* ethical issues, *recognizing* misunderstandings, and *bringing* new information to light. I find that bit-by-bit, piece-by-piece, each voice draws a wider and broader picture.

The results of ethical case conferences should not be predetermined but rather *flow* from the participation of the members of the group. Any changes in the direction of care are solely the responsibility of the physician and patient/surrogate and are agreed on in private *after* the conference.

Before the meeting:
- *I review the case with fresh eyes and ears* looking for buried clues that can answer questions regarding our patient's desires.
- Although it is often not possible, try to *meet* with the family before the meeting and prepare them for what will take place.

At the meeting I:

WE CAN, BUT SHOULD WE?

- *Explain* to the group that the purpose of the meeting is to allow everyone to share their own values and thoughts with the other members with the hope of arriving at an understanding about what the patient would want done if he or she was able to speak.
- *Point out* that all therapeutic decisions are solely those of the patient's surrogate and physician, not those of the group.
- *Remember* the patient's values come first and list what are known about them.
- *Explore* other issues that are most likely involved such as family dynamics, cultural, spiritual, educational, or financial considerations.
- *Determine* what questions are being asked, who is asking them, and what might be behind these questions.
- *Obtain* facts and information from many angles: medical, social, financial, legal, and spiritual.
- *Explain* this information when there is confusion.

Some of the most important things for medical personnel to recognize when dealing with a patient who has a serious illness are:

- What it is we need to *know?*
- What questions need to be *asked?*
- How do we *teach ourselves not to be afraid* to ask the hard questions?
- How can we *identify where we can find* the answers to these questions

We should avoid the pitfalls that are unfortunately all too common because of:

- Using *medical jargon.*
- Over *simplifying.*
- *Forcing* our own viewpoint.
- *Ignoring* patient values.
- *Frightening* the patient in order for them to make a decision.

Time and motivation make it difficult for the physicians and staff to learn the techniques of active listening. At the very least, the

135

facilitator of a multidisciplinary patient conference should have training in this important form of communication. In a conference setting, a trained facilitator can help smooth the ruffled feathers of families and staff by following these active listening techniques[9]:

- *Pay attention* to the environment. Is it inclusive and comfortable?
- *Be patient* and present to the speaker.
- *Let* the speaker know that you have heard him with appropriate eye contact and body language.
- *Do not allow* one individual to control the discussion.
- *Stop crosstalk.* One person speaks at a time.
- *Be compassionate* and empathetic as you listen.
- *Listen* with an open mind.
- *Disregard* your agenda.
- *Pause* before speaking and speak slowly.
- *Ask* for clarification
- *Don't assume* your words are understood.

Active listening with empathy, flexibility, and experience is important for a peaceful, open ended, exchange of information to take place between the hospital staff, the patient, and family.

---

1. Chapter 1: *Living Life on the Edge* (Autonomy)
2. Chapter 2: *Changing Image* (Beneficence)
3. Chapter 3: *Not a Leg to Stand On* (Non-maleficence)
4. Chapter 4: *The Shadow Side* (Justice)
5. Chapter 5: *The Small Card* (Fidelity)
6. Chapter 7: *Window of Opportunity* (Capacity)
7. Chapter 8: *Who's On First?* (Surrogacy)
8. Chapter 11: *"I Love My Son"* (Case Conferences)
9. Taken in part and revised from Lindahl, Kay "Listening: A Sacred Art and Spiritual Practice." *Presence*: (December 2014) pages 19-26. Courtesy of Kay Lindahl www.sacredlistening.com

18
The Last Word

It is sobering to contemplate a loved one dying. Most often we are reminded of our own mortality; living and dying are just a veil away. We feel the fragility of life and wonder what our last breath would be like.

Great minds have pondered the meanings of life and death through art and writing. My father, Sidney M. Gospe, M.D., was an obstetrician in San Francisco. He often told me, *We begin to die from the moment of our conception.* From his wisdom, I have come to honor the sacredness of both the birthing and the dying process as one part of our human experience.

The image of a doctor as healer in *The Doctor*[1], a painting by Sir Luke Fields in 1891, has been a guiding metaphor for me. A late Nineteenth Century physician, Sir James Watson, is at the bedside of a young girl. The girl's parents keep vigil without ceasing. Her mother sits at a table, sobbing as she buries her head in her arms. Her father is filled with sorrow as he stands at the child's bedside. He watches the physician for signs of hope and prays for a miracle. The doctor sits, leaning forward, one hand under his chin, as if he searches the wealth of his experience for a way to help his patient. Perhaps, he prays for a healing miracle to manifest itself in the hours to come. Or he meets a familiar feeling of inadequacy. Dr. Watson waits for the outcome, as do the parents.

The painting reminds me of the powerful responsibility that families place in their physician, especially when there is no medication, procedure, or test that can reverse the coming potential of death. The physician's compassionate presence at his patient's bedside speaks volumes even when there is nothing left to do except to wait for the eventual ending: recovery or death.

I met a similar experience when I was a medical intern in Minneapolis. I remember that frigid, snow-covered winter night when I made an ambulance call to a bungalow tucked away in a quiet neighborhood. My driver and I entered the home. It was eerily silent. Two firemen nodded to us at the doorway and pointed the way to the nursery. There, a young couple bent over their infant daughter who lay motionless in her crib. The parents' stunned faces radiated both hope and fear.

I felt the presence of death in the room. The baby's face was ashen. Her body appeared frozen to her crib. I knew the infant was dead. In my heart, I felt hopeless, at a loss for words. Both mother and father waited beside me in silence, hoping against hope that I could make everything right.

I was unable to speak. I felt I was moving in slow motion as I began my physical examination. There were no signs of life when I placed my stethoscope on her cooling body. A pink baby blanket lay close by. Gently, reverently, I picked it up and covered the babe's body and face. Her parents began to sob. Teardrops moistened the eyes of the two burly firemen as well as my own.

That night, I learned a physician was not just one who examines a body, writes a prescription, and orders a test. That one simple action with a tiny blanket taught me that a symbol can speak volumes. The emotion in the room moved me so much that I don't remember what I said or did.

Words often paint pictures as vivid as those created by Da Vinci or Rembrandt. In 1916, the Bengali poet, Tagore, wrote the following in his poem *Stray Birds*[2]:

> *Let life be as beautiful as summer flowers*
> *And death as beautiful as autumn leaves.*

These few words remind me of the role nature plays in my own life. For me, I hope I will not fear my death as it approaches. Rather, I want to accept it as a vital part of my own cycle of existence. I have been privileged to witness the beauty encircling many of my patients who were comfortable as they accepted the coming of their death. Their examples will guide me as I, too, near the end of my own life.

I have experienced a steady evolution since my first day at Stanford Medical School in September of 1959. As a young physician, I thought of myself as being a goal-oriented scientist with a strong desire to *find the problem and fix it*. I likened myself as a pit bull with the patients' symptoms a bone in my mouth. The tension carried in my jaws remained until I discovered a diagnosis and treatment.

Over the years, I grew to realize that all of us are unique human beings. We are all wise, complex, and filled with hopes and dreams. Within our hearts we know the right thing to do, to say, to be. Our patients are far more than a collection of symptoms awaiting a diagnosis and specific treatment.

I have learned to listen to my intuition, that nudge that can guide me through difficult spaces. I urge you to take notice as a caregiver and/or family member. When you sense that something doesn't feel right, this may be a warning sign to examine the situation further, to investigate, to ask for clarification. When brought out in the open, there is a good chance that new information may reverse your discomfort and solve an important issue or reveal necessary information. And when there is nothing to do, or no words come, wait in silence and pause in the moment.

My wish is that this small book has offered you some insight with tools to help you in your pursuit of the incurable condition called life.

---

1. Fields, Sir Luke, *The Doctor, 1891:* The Tate Museum, London
2. Tagore, Rabindranath. *Stray Birds*, Macmillan Company 1916: Stanza 82

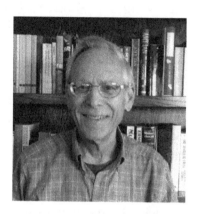

About the Author

J. Michael Gospe, M.D. joined Santa Rosa Memorial Hospital's newly formed bioethics group in 1982 and became its chairperson the two years later. In 1999, upon retiring from his twenty-nine-year practice in gastroenterology and internal medicine, he established the role of Medical Director of Ethics at the hospital. He continues to hold both positions at the time of this book's completion.

Dr. Gospe has consulted on more than a thousand patients with medical ethical issues. Many patients and their families have inspired him by their love of life and their acceptance of the unfolding of their last days. Others have saddened him by the paralyzing fear that ruled their final hours. Working within this field of *end of life decisions,* Dr. Gospe has deepened his awareness of the complexity and beauty of the human spirit. He has written this book in order to enable healthcare providers and families to better support patients and loved ones as they journey through the closing chapter of their lives.

Also by
J. Michael Gospe, M.D.

<u>Memoirs</u>

Illuminations in an Elevator: Evolution of a Physician

Images from Childhood

<u>Biographical Novel</u>

Lady in Black: A Woman's Journey

Available at
https://gospemedicalethics.wordpress.com/home/